LOCKDOWN 2020
COVID-19 IN UK

KEN MENON

authorHOUSE

AuthorHouse™ UK
1663 Liberty Drive
Bloomington, IN 47403 USA
www.authorhouse.co.uk
Phone: UK TFN: 0800 0148641 (Toll Free inside the UK)
   UK Local: 02036 956322 (+44 20 3695 6322 from outside the UK)

© 2020 Ken Menon. All rights reserved.

The Holy Bible, Berean Study Bible, BSB
Copyright ©2016 by Bible Hub
Used by Permission. All Rights Reserved Worldwide.

No part of this book may be reproduced, stored in a retrieval system, or transmitted by any means without the written permission of the author.

Published by AuthorHouse 10/06/2020

ISBN: 978-1-6655-8037-3 (sc)
ISBN: 978-1-6655-8038-0 (hc)
ISBN: 978-1-6655-8036-6 (e)

Print information available on the last page.

Any people depicted in stock imagery provided by Getty Images are models,
and such images are being used for illustrative purposes only.
Certain stock imagery © Getty Images.

This book is printed on acid-free paper.

Because of the dynamic nature of the Internet, any web addresses or links contained in this book may have changed since publication and may no longer be valid. The views expressed in this work are solely those of the author and do not necessarily reflect the views of the publisher, and the publisher hereby disclaims any responsibility for them.

This book is dedicated to the memory of Dr.Li Wenliang who alerted the world to the presence of the coronavirus infection, now known as Covid-19

He died of Covid-19

'Greater love has no one than this, that he lay down his life for his friends'
John 15:13 BSB

CONTENTS

The Scene	1
Anatomy of a disaster	34
Barbed wire disease	65
Collateral damage	87
'The Good, The Bad, The Ugly'	107
Release	159
Death and Debt	189
Aftermath	196
'This is war'	230
Abbreviations	233

THE SCENE

Human history is littered with stories of epidemics, pandemics and pestilence which killed many and decimated populations. Typhoid fever was so severe in Athens in 435 BC that it killed many including the leader at the time; the soldier, politician and orator, Pericles. There were two additional waves of the plague - in 429 BC and in the 427-426 BC winter. So many were killed that the germ did not have sufficient numbers of people left through which to spread; the epidemic died out. The Athenian historian Thucydides described the plague as having such a catastrophic effect that people did not comply with any law as they did not see any future for themselves. People expected life was likely to be short due to the epidemic. People lived as if they were under a under a life sentence.

Covid-19 would not be the last. It is caused by one of a family of viruses called coronaviruses. 'Corona' comes from the Latin word meaning a crown. The crown is made of particles of the virus like bulbs which protrude from the surface of the virus. Some describe the virus as resembling the solar corona on the surface of the sun.

On 31st December 2019 China informed the World Health Organisation (WHO) office in the country about cases of pneumonia in Wuhan. They did not know the cause of the chest infection. Wuhan is the capital city of Hubei province which is in Central China. Wuhan has a population of about 11 million people which makes it ninth in terms of size of population in cities of China. It is an important place of culture, economics and politically. It is designated as a National Central City.

The late Chairman Mao-Tse- Tsung (Mao Zedong) had his villa, Meiling Buildings, in Wuhan.

Then on 3rd January 2020 there were 44 cases of pneumonia. Some of the patients worked in the seafood market in Huanan which is located in Wuhan. There was no evidence at this stage of human to human transmission of infection. Based on the information available to it, WHO did not advice any travel restrictions to China.

The seafood market in Huanan, also known as the Huanan Wholesale Seafood Market is large, covering an area of about 50,000 square metres, which is about the size of seven football fields. When it opened over 10 years ago it had 400 stalls and this had grown to 1000 stalls at the time of its closure by the Chinese authorities in January 2020. Seafood is brought to the market in water tanks which makes the market wet. Fish is not the only food sold there. Various types of animal flesh are available. The choice of flesh is extensive and includes rats, camels, dogs, beavers, foxes, peacocks, pheasant, snakes etc. One particular snake is the Chinese krait or Taiwanese krait. This snake which belongs to the zoological family elapidae is common in Asia. It reaches a length of 3-5 feet and is venomous. Its bite releases a neurotoxin (nerve poison) which can cause paralysis. Untreated, about a quarter of human victims of the bite of this snake could die.

The market was said to have been officially inspected by the authorities and passed as satisfactory in 2019.

Animals are packed close by to each other and are often slaughtered and skinned in the market. Dead and live animals are visible side by a side. The age of meat for sale is often unknown. A user of the WeChat messaging service wrote that in 2013 stale prawns from the market were sold to local restaurants. In 2017 fish sold in two of the stalls were contaminated with a chemical called malachite green. Malachite green is used as a dye and as an antibiotic for fish. It is known to cause lung and liver tumours in rats in very large doses. It is unlikely that any significant amounts are consumed by humans.

Wet markets are not unique to China and are found in other parts of Asia.

In January 2020 the Chinese government said that trade in and consumption of wild animals would be banned in China.

Part of the reason for Chinese liking of food is because starvation is deeply ingrained in the national psyche. The famine in the years of rule by President Mao Zedong compelled people to eat whatever that was available to alleviate hunger. Another reason for wanting wild life is the health beliefs of many Chinese people.

How did Chinese start eating wild animals? The answer to this partly lies in the policy called the Great Leap. This was an economic policy introduced by Mao Zedong which lasted from 1958 to 1962. The purpose of the Great Leap was to transform the agrarian economy of China. People were forced to work in communes. Farmers had to meet quotas of production, which often could not be met. Starvation ensued. Almost 50 million people died. When Hebei and Shandong provinces banned the consumption of meat, Mao Zedong said 'this is good, why can the whole country not do the same; we should eat less'. He advocated a firm and ruthless approach. He maintained that when there is not enough to eat people starved to death and that it was better for half of the people to die so that the other half 'can eat their fill'.

As far as grain harvests were concerned Chairman Mao maintained that the Party act with speed in gathering grain before farmers could lay their hands on it.

The whole of the Chinese Communist Party (CCP) operated then as now, on a hierarchical system. In this arrangement the higher one was in the line, the more one was entitled to in terms of food, cigarettes etc. Of course at the top of the pinnacle was Chairman Mao who lived in apparent grandeur. While people in the countryside and farms starved, Party cadres enjoyed unlimited supplies of food and cigarettes. Frank Dikotter describes how at one four day conference 260 cadres ate 210kg of beef, 500kg of pork. 680 chickens, 40kg of ham, 150 litres of wine and smoked 79 cartons of cigarettes.

Children sometimes starved to death because adults stole rations designated for children in kindergartens and schools.

People ate leaves and bark from trees and even soil and mud to combat hunger. Leather from chairs was cut into small pieces, soaked and eaten.

Whatever that was available to eat, was eaten, even dead comrades. The fear of starvation is real and may provide an explanation for their liking of wild animals for food.

In Wuhan in 1959 food poisoning was a frequent occurrence. It occurred because of poor hygiene. Vats of food due for market had broken seals allowing worms to contaminate them. Maggots were found in food. Rotten eggs were used in cakes and workers urinated on the floor. Sanitation was poor and food was often rotten.

Epidemics have occurred throughout human history. Covid-19 is often compared with the Spanish flu of 1918. It is useful to look at what happened during the Spanish flu. That global pandemic lasted for two years and was caused by, what is called the H1N1 influenza virus. The next time H1N1 appeared was in 2009 as swine flu. Despite its name, Spanish flu did not originate in Spain. It spread to Spain from France. The first wave was not particularly bad and was like the usual winter flu. The infection rate dropped during the summer of 1918. But after this apparent calm came the storm - it is as if the virus underwent a change or mutation to become severe and virulent. From September until November 2019 many people died from the virus. Troop movements at the end of World War 1 caused deaths of large numbers of apparently healthy young men and women. Death was caused by pneumonia, blisters and bleeding from the nose and the lungs, which filled with fluid. The lungs became so congested with fluid that it caused patients to 'drown' in their own secretions. We now know that this extreme reaction to the virus is called super- or hyper-inflammation or a cytokine storm. This is seen in some patients with the current coronavirus infection or Covid-19.

There was then a third wave of the Spanish flu virus which affected Australia, from where it made its way back to Europe. Death from the third wave was as high as that during the second wave. The third wave occurred in the winter of 1918 and ended in the summer of 1919. By this time the virus appears to have subsided and the epidemic had run its course. The author John M.Barry wrote that the flu "made the entire world a killing zone". The Spanish flu pandemic affected a quarter of the world's population of 2 billion, meaning that 500 million had the flu. Of this up to 100 million died. China was not particularly severely affected by the Spanish flu pandemic although some believe that the virus may have originated in China. However there is no conclusive evidence to support such a hypothesis.

This is a brief description of the magnitude of the problem the country and the world are now facing with Covid-19, despite all the advances in medical science since 1918.

The SARS (Severe Acute Respiratory Syndrome) epidemic which lasted from 2002-2004 originated in China. It spread from south China to Hong Kong and thereafter to the rest of the world. It affected about 8000 people across the world and about 800 died. The epidemic lasted about 4 months and was brought under control by effective public health measures. SARS is Severe Acute Respiratory Syndrome caused by a coronavirus. It is similar to what we are experiencing with Covid-19 at present and carried a severe risk to health and of death.

The SARS outbreak started on 16th November 2002 in Guandong province in southern China. It is a large province bordering Hong Kong and with a population of about 115 million people. The infection mainly affected farmers and restaurant workers. But as patients were admitted to hospitals healthcare workers were increasingly affected. The Chinese government prevented the press from publishing information about the epidemic and even prevented its citizens outside the province from being informed about the outbreak of the infection. The WHO was notified about the outbreak of the infection only on 10th February 2003, almost three months after the beginning of the epidemic. WHO officials who visited China were prevented from going to Guandong. Following much international criticism China agreed to change the way it notified the WHO. Covid-19 has shown that nothing has changed.

The virus that caused SARS was identified in cave-dwelling bats with civets acting as a kind of 'middleman' in transfer of the virus. Civets are carnivorous mammals that have been variously described as looking like cats, mongoose, ferrets etc. Civets are common in Asia and often have their own local names. For eg in Sri Lanka it is called 'uguduwa'. Surprisingly the epidemic lasted only about five months and vanished. While the subsidence of SARS provided relief to peoples, governments and health systems, it raised the question as to what happened to the virus. Would it raise its head again! Would it be more severe if it reappeared? At its peak the Chinese government threatened to execute any person who violated the quarantine that was imposed to help combat the infection! This sounds similar to what the President of the Philippines said recently about lockdown in that country, when he ordered shoot to kill. At the time, a physician, Dr. Jiang Yanyong sent a letter to TV stations in China and Hong Kong stating that China was concealing the true extent of the infection in the mainland. It does not appear that the contents of this letter was aired on TV. However the letter had leaked to other news organisations. Dr. Jian Yanyong and his wife were arrested and eventually released in July 2004. In 2004 Dr. Jiang Yanyong was awarded the Ramon Magsaysay award for revealing the truth about the SARS epidemic and for his help in dealing with the epidemic. The award is made in memory of a past President of the Philippines, Ramon Magsaysay, for 'courageous public service'.

In the SARS epidemic there was concealment of what was happening in China and delay in informing authorities both within China and the WHO about the emerging illness. This delayed global information and action to combat the infection. However, public health measures that were instituted at the time helped to contain the spread of infection. Hong Kong for example was particularly badly affected. In Hong Kong hand-washing was encouraged, masks were worn and schools were closed.

The manner in which SARS was concealed by China is similar to what the world experienced with Covid-19 in 2020. There does not appear to be any change in the approach by the Chinese to dealing with or alerting the world community early, about the emerging risks to world health. This could become a continuing issue with the large reservoir of coronaviruses in bats in for e.g. Guangdong province.

The SARS virus called SARS-CoV-1 and the current Covid-19 virus called SARS-CoV-2 are closely related. Both of them originated in bats and their genetic structure or genome are 80% identical. This not surprising as viruses are related, like man is related to chimpanzees where 98% of the genome is identical between the two. Marilyn J. Roossinck, Professor of Plant Pathology and Environmental Microbiology, Pennsylvania State University calls SARS-Cov1 and SARS-Cov2 the 'killing cousins'. SARS was more lethal but Covid-19 spreads much faster. Therefore Covid-19 has the far greater potential to lead to death, as we are witnessing in countries around the world.

In February 2020 President Xi Jinping of China said that it was vital to contain the Covid-19 virus. He also warned against any cover-ups similar to what happened with SARS in 2002. The Central Political and Legal Affairs Commission in China wrote "Anyone who puts the face of politicians before the interests of the people will be the sinner of a millennium, to the party and the people". It continued, "Anyone who deliberately delays and hides the reporting of cases out of his or her own self-interest will be nailed on the pillar of shame for eternity."

Swine flu was the next pandemic in recent times. It occurred in 2009 and lasted for about a year. Swine flu was caused by the H1N1 virus which occurs in pigs and from where transmission to humans occurred. Transmission of a virus from an animal to humans is called a zoonosis; hence swine flu is a zoonotic flu. Swine flu affected about 10% of the world population, which was 6.5 billion people at the time. About 700 million persons were affected and 150,000 to 180,000 people died form it worldwide. H1N1 caused the pandemic of Spanish flu in 1918. There were reports that the epidemic may have been caused by a leak of the virus from a laboratory. The genetic material of H1N1 was made up of that from normal human flu virus, a bird flu virus and virus in pigs. The virus was in Mexico and was identified in 2009 as causing swine flu.

Following this epidemic UK Department of Health reviewed its plans to deal with any future outbreaks and thereby to help the NHS better deal with any future outbreak of illness. One of the key aspects of the plan was to try and contain any future epidemic by identifying persons who are infected and by isolating and treating them. By doing these it was thought the spread in the community could be curtailed. The Influenza Pandemic Preparedness Strategy 2011 document implies that the UK would not be able to contain an influenza virus if it came to the UK. Therefore isolation and curtailment of spread are vital.

In the 2003 SARS epidemic the UK was able to identify and isolate patients. These two steps probably helped to limit the spread of the virus. But this was a virus that did not spread as rapidly as the current Covid-19 virus does. Would the preventive measures used in 2003 have worked in 2020? We know that testing and isolation of infected persons would have helped to slow the rate of transmission of Covid-19, despite its rapid rate of spread. The containment strategy alone was not likely to work. It may have worked with a rigid containment method which limited the continued entry of the virus into the UK.

Then in 2012 came MERS (Middle East Respiratory Syndrome).

This too was caused by a coronavirus, called MERS-Cov, which first appeared in Saudi Arabia. In fact, most of the cases of MERV were in the Arabian region. But the infection was also reported in people in Europe (France, Germany, Netherlands, Greece, Italy, UK etc), US, China and the Republic of Korea. It was reported that up to one third of patients who got MERV died from the disease. In the UK there were four cases of MERV of which three patients died. The source of the MERV virus is thought to be camels. Like the current advice, people were advised about regular hand washing. They were also advised to avoid camel meat, camel milk and any form of raw food that could have been contaminated with animal secretions. MERS was not as infectious as Covid-19. It also did not appear to pass from person to person as quickly or as easily as Covid-19 does.

MERS occurred 10 years after SARS and both were due to coronaviruses which had come from animals. There was now enough information to show that transmission of coronaviruses to humans was not unusual. Such animal to human transmission of coronavirus is likely to be a recurring event. This was a wakeup call which does not appear to have been sufficiently heeded, given that a scientific paper in 2017 published that 'coronaviruses are capable of mutating (*changing*) at high frequency'... 'which can lead to possible future outbreaks in humans'. Coronaviruses cause infections in many species of animals and in human beings, in whom until recently they usually caused mild upper respiratory infections like the common cold and fever with a dry cough. These were self-limiting symptoms which usually resolved without the need for medical attention. The evolution of viruses shows that even the virus causing the common cold or coryza may have crossed from bats to human beings in the last 200 years or so. Coryza is now a frequent occurrence because the virus is endemic and lives among humans, usually causing symptoms which seldom are more than a nuisance.

Now in 2020 we see the transfer of yet another coronavirus, Covid-19, to humans, on a larger and likely to be a significantly lethal scale.

In addition to the various forms of viral influenza epidemics, another threat to health in the UK was posed by Bovine Spongiform Encephalopathy (BSE) or 'mad cow disease' in the 1980's. The disease occurred in cattle which had been infected by an abnormal protein called a prion. This caused damage to the nervous system of cattle (a neuro-degenerative disease). Cattle got the disease by eating offal from other cattle which had died from the disease. It also occurred because cattle were fed flesh and offal from sheep that were infected with a disease called scrapie. Scrapie is also a nerve degenerating or nerve-damaging disease caused by prion. Humans got the prion by eating contaminated beef and meat products. This caused a similar damage and degeneration of the nervous system in humans called Creutzfeld- Jacob disease (CJD). CJD took years to develop in an affected human being and caused behaviour and personality problems, difficulty with coordination etc. Most patients died within 18 months of the onset of symptoms. CJD was not like Covid-19; it could not be transmitted from person to person by contact or secretions.

Prions are abnormal proteins where their chemical structure is misfolded. The damage this causes to the three-dimensional structure of the protein is supposed to endow it with 'infectious' ability. It does so by causing protein molecules that are in close proximity to it to become misfolded themselves. The term prion comes from 'proteinaceous infected particle'. Prions can cause degeneration of the nervous system in animals and humans.

At that time of CJD the government of the day assured the public that British beef was safe to eat. This was based on the assumption that meat and meat products from BSE infected cattle would not infect other animals. This was an erroneous assertion; cats were found to get the disease. This meant that cats had acquired the disease after having eating infected beef or beef products. The exports of British beef declined with a ban on export being imposed by the European Union.

A subsequent inquiry in to the BSE crisis showed that the government had been slow to respond in its communication with the public and in how it dealt with the crisis. About four and a half million cattle were eventually slaughtered in the UK. More worrying is that we do not know how many people are still carrying the prion and how many of these people would, in the future, develop symptoms and be diagnosed with CJD. All cattle born or imported to the UK after 1st July 1996 now have a cattle passport which helps to keep track of an animal from birth to death. This would help in the future if there was any infection or disease that may be linked to cattle.

What has never been explained is why cattle that are herbivores were fed meet and offal. This had the effect of converting herbivores to carnivores.

The pursuit of profit inflicted great harm on the farming industry and on the health of the public.

What is the relevance of CJD to Covid19, one may ask? Simply put, government policy must always be to act in time and speedily and to always seek to protect the public.

The World Health Organisation (WHO) has a vital part to play in the health of people throughout the world. It is the custodian of global health, monitoring outbreaks of disease, identifying risks to people and to their communities and countries. It provides guidance and support in managing threats to public health. To help in discharging its wide remit, the WHO depends on information shared with it by each and every country that is a member of WHO. Important surveillance information about epidemics and other risks to public health are collated by WHO, analysed and in turn shared with its members. It leaves each individual member country to deal with the information that it sends out, in the best way that a country considers. This would take into account local factors, resources, manpower, culture etc. Most countries look to the WHO for information and guidance because of the wealth of skills and experience that it has in dealing with medical crises. Therefore the WHO is a guardian of the world's health.

When the United Nations came into existence after World War 2 it decided to set up a global health organisation. WHO came into being in 1948 on the founding principle that 'health is a human right and all people should enjoy the highest standard of health'. The purpose of the WHO as stated in its constitution are:

i. 'to act as the directing and co-ordinating authority on international health work'
ii. 'to stimulate and advance work to eradicate epidemic, endemic and other diseases'

The WHO vision is 'of a world in which all peoples attain the highest possible level of health, and our mission to promote health, keep the world safe and serve the vulnerable, with measurable impact for people at country level. We are individually and collectively committed to put these values into practice'.

Yet it is important to realise that the WHO is at the same time a 'quasi-political' organisation. It is not only an independent health organisation. It is the voice of its constituent members and as such 'might is right'. The heavyweights in the organisation could influence its decisions in a subtle, discreet way. They in effect pay the piper! None of this means that it is a political organisation in the sense that it is openly manipulated for political ends or that it has a political office; far from it. But it is susceptible to pressure from countries at times of crises. But these are the very times when the independence of the WHO is most needed.

Working for the eradication of infectious diseases has been the WHO's greatest achievement in its history. Elimination of smallpox and to a very large extent poliomyelitis worldwide is commendable. Couple these achievements with its campaigns on vaccination and one readily sees that the WHO is a force for good in the world. It has worked hard to reduce infant and child mortality and its preventive work on tobacco control, especially given entrenched commercial interests, have to be lauded. More recently its work on family planning and birth control and on the prevention and management of non- communicable diseases (NCD) like diabetes and heart disease are successful, leading to increased survival and reduced human suffering. However the WHO is a slow moving bureaucracy and increasingly susceptible to political influences.

Take the example of the recent Ebola crisis in Africa between 2014 and 2016 which mainly affected Sierra Leone, Liberia and Guinea with respective case fatality rates of 28%, 45% and 67%. Over 28,000 people were infected and more than 11,000 died. Following the epidemic WHO came under intense scrutiny for the way it had handled the epidemic. Experts from Harvard Global Health Institute and the London School of Tropical Medicine and Hygiene said that there needed to be 'greater transparency and accountability and the WHO should be required to respond to freedom of information requests'. But what is most relevant in the current context is the report's recommendation that 'WHO should promote early reporting of outbreaks by commending countries that rapidly and publicly share information, while publishing lists of countries that delay reporting.' While the WHO knew that there was an Ebola epidemic developing and that it was spreading, it did not raise an alarm early enough. If the other recommendations of the report had been acted upon the world may just have witnessed an attenuated spread of Covid-19 and with this an accompanying reduced global death rate. Specifically the report recommended that there be a dedicated centre for outbreak response and that 'a transparent and politically protected WHO Standing Emergency Committee should be delegated with the responsibility for declaring public health emergencies.' Health experts called for better leadership. Sir Jeremy Farrar, the director of the Welcome Trust, said: "Today's report includes some sobering lessons and sets out critical recommendations for increasing our resilience to future epidemics. Particularly welcome are the calls for greater investment from governments to build a core capacity to detect, report and respond rapidly to outbreaks. "It's vital that the lessons learned are translated into concrete action if we are to avert another crisis on the scale of Ebola." Jeremy Farrar wrote for e.g. about the local office in Brazzaville, the capital of the Republic of Congo, as 'riven by politics, corruption and endemic weak leadership.' Writing about the Ebola epidemic Prof Peter Piot, the director of the London School of Hygiene and Tropical Medicine, said '"Major reform of national and global systems to respond to epidemics are not only feasible, but also essential, so that we do not witness such depths of suffering, death and social and economic havoc in future epidemics. ' The recommended independent Standing Committee was not established and the benefits that may have accrued from it were not available during the outbreak of Covid-19.The failure or inability to respond early enough in 2020 is a near identical re-run of events in Africa with the Ebola epidemics. The paper 'Ten essential reforms before the next pandemic. The report of the Harvard-LSHTM Independent Panel on the Global Response to Ebola' published in Lancet in November 2015 is doubly sobering today. It shows at best the incompetence at the heart of the WHO and at worst its callous irresponsibility towards world health. Ebola was an opportunity for the WHO to change; but it failed!

The words of Sir Jeremy Farrar are particularly relevant to what probably happened at the outset with Convid-19. Would the world have been better prepared if, at least, the reporting ability of the WHO was robust and independent of interference, as has been suggested in some quarters? The Report of the Ebola Interim Assessment Panel of July 2015 stated 'The Panel firmly believes that this is a defining moment not only for WHO and the global health emergency response but also for the governance of the entire global health system'. The casual reader may ask what has changed since then.

As far as the UK and most countries are concerned these statements should have carried some significance. We should have been wary of pronouncements by the WHO, especially about infections originating in China. The UK government and its scientific experts should have been aware of China being 'economical with the acualite', and of the WHO's tardiness of response.

On 22 January the WHO met at its Strategic Health Operations Centre (SHOC) in Geneva to consider whether to declare the coronavirus infection a 'Public Health Emergency of International Concern' (PHEIC). This would be a red flag or alert to the countries of the world of an emerging epidemic or pandemic. This would sound a call to action by countries to take appropriate steps to mitigate the effects of the virus in its citizens. Firstly, there were submissions at the meeting from China, Japan and Thailand, where there had been cases of the infection. This was followed by contributions by the fifteen members and six advisors of the emergency committee. These are people with skills, knowledge and experience from around the world. The main issues being discussed was whether person-to-person transmission of the virus could take place and how easily this could happen. If this was so, then it is a grave threat to world health and immediate action would have been called for. Opinion was divided on the matter; a unanimous decision would clear the path to declare a world-wide emergency.

As there was no agreement in the group, The Director General of the WHO, Dr.Tedros Adhanom Ghebreyesus, suspended the meeting for a few more days. But at this second meeting there was yet no agreement. China opposed declaring an emergency at the meeting of 22nd January. It could not have acted alone at this stage because the other members of the committee were from the USA, Thailand, Russia, France, South Korea, Canada, Japan, Netherlands, Australia, Senegal, Singapore, Saudi Arabia, Sweden, and New Zealand. For the vote to have been split at this stage, there is no doubt that many in the group were not convinced that there was a threat to public health.

The meeting was adjourned yet again with a recall of the group at short notice if events on the ground changed. Finally on 30th January WHO declared the pandemic as a PHEIC.

In April 2020 US President, Donald Trump accused the WHO of covering up information about the spread of coronavirus and of placing political correctness above the lives of people. He was scathing about the handling of the pandemic by the WHO and threatened to withhold funding for it. The US contributes $500 million annually to the WHO while China contributes $30 million. He insisted that the WHO 'must be held accountable'.

Where in China the Covid-19 virus originated from continues to be surrounded in mystery and confusion compounded by limited information. Whether it arose from animals in the market or in the Wuhan Institute of Virology is still a source of much speculation. The Institute is where research had been going on about viruses and especially viruses in bats. A scientist in the Institute, Dr.Shi Zhengli, had been conducting research into deadly coronaviruses found in bats. It is interesting that one of these viruses has a genetic code which is 96% identical to the genetic code of Covid-19. The Chinese authorities maintain that no virus could have escaped from the research laboratories as they have a high level of bio-security. Laboratories around the world which deal with deadly germs have very high levels of security to protect those who work in them and the public, from accidental contamination with or escape of germs. Escape of any germs outside the confines of a laboratory is serious; they could cause infections and spread widely and even cross national boundaries.

We know that many scientists across the world and in the WHO maintain that there is no convincing evidence that Covid-19 came from the laboratory in Wuhan. However there have been concerns about safety at the institute. A deputy director at the Institute had expressed concerns in 2019 about safety there. A senior Communist Party member at the Institute, Professor Yuan, also said in 2019 that maintenance at the Institute had been neglected, due to limited funding. Yuan Zhimimg who was head of bio-security wrote about serious concerns related to bio-security and stated that 'maintenance cost is generally neglected' and that the laboratory was run on 'minimal operational costs or none at all'. The laboratory was constructed with help from France and has bio-security level 4. He said that there was a need for bio-safety at the Institute to be improved. However the same person commented in April 2020 that it was malicious to say that the virus originated in the Institute. When the pandemic occurred and there was speculation about the origin of the virus, Professor Yuan claimed that what was written was rumour which had been 'pulled out of thin air'.

In January 2018 US scientists who had visited the Wuhan laboratory were concerned about safety in the laboratory. Of course there is no direct causal link between less than ideal bio-security in the Institute and the spread of coronavirus.

Researchers from South China University of Technology published a paper on 6th February 2020 concluding that "the killer coronavirus probably originated from a laboratory in Wuhan. Safety level at the Institute may need to be reinforced in high-risk biohazards laboratories". The paper was withdrawn, although no one refuted the findings expressed in it.

In 2002 WHO had expressed concern regarding bio-security in the Chinese National Institute of Bio-security in Beijing. This followed cases of SARS. Instead of having a bios-security level of 3 (BSL3) the laboratory had a BSL2 status. In Wuhan the laboratory had BSL4 but was known to have poorly applied policies and procedures.

Bio-security levels are also known as bio-safety levels and pathogen protection levels. These are a set of security levels applied to laboratories working with germs, bacteria, viruses etc. The purpose of these levels is to ensure safety for the workers and for the wider community by containing germs within the facility and preventing accidental contamination of the community outside the confines of the facility. There are usually four levels of bio-security. BSL3 and BSL4 involve extremely rigid safety standards involving use of bio-security suits, clean insured air, air circulation and extraction etc to prevent even the slightest possibility of escape of a germ.

Some of the pictures that the world has seen of Wuhan Institute of Virology show the door in one of the refrigerators broken. These pictures have since been deleted. It is known that US diplomats were concerned about security in the Institute and warned the US State Department of the risk of another 'SARS- like epidemic'.

It was and still is important for China to be more transparent in what happened in the early days prior to the pandemic being declared. The French President, Emmanuel Macron said that what happened is not known. The Chinese Embassy in London maintained 'there has never been any cover up, nor was a cover-up ever allowed to happen'.

It is interesting to note at this stage that the US National Institutes of Health had funded the study on bats at the Wuhan laboratory. The US government provided a grant of $3.7 million to the Institute in Wuhan to study bats. In2017 a scientific paper in the journal PLOS Pathogens was published jointly by Dr. Shi Zhengli, Peter Daszak and others with the title 'Discovery of a rich gene pool of bat SARS- related coronaviruses provides new insights into the origin of SARS coronavirus'. The authors wrote *'we have provided sufficient evidence to conclude that SARS-CoV most likely originated from horseshoe bats…the risk of spillover into people and emergence of a disease similar to SARS is possible…. Thus, we propose that monitoring of SARS related-CoV evolution at this and other sites should continue, as well as examination of human behavioural risk for infection ………., to determine if spill-over is already occurring at these sites and to design intervention strategies to avoid future disease* emergence.

The paper states *'diverse SARS-CoVs capable of direct transmission to humans are circulating in bats in this cave. Our current study therefore offers a clearer picture on the evolutionary origin of SARS-CoV and highlights the risk of future emergence of SARS-like diseases.*

Here we encounter a clear pointer to the possibility of transmission of viruses from bats to humans.

Another scientific paper published in the scientific journal Nature, stated that transmission of viruses from wildlife is a risk to animals and humans. Bats are recognised as the source of most coronaviruses. These viruses transferred from bats to humans caused SARS. The same mode of transmission occurred with Covid-19.

In 2018 Dr.Devi Sridhar, Professor of Global Public Health in the University of Edinburgh had said that a virus might jump species to humans and spread worldwide causing a pandemic.

Opinions vary as to whether the virus originated from the Wuhan wet market after it had leaked from the Wuhan laboratory.

Scientists from the University of North Carolina and from the WIV concluded from their joint work that the original SARS virus could cross from bats to human beings. They continued to work with viruses and genetically altered bat cornaviruses producing a chimera virus. This virus was found to be highly pathogenic, implying that the virus could affect humans easily and that there was no treatment if it did so.

Could the virus really be a genetically modified virus? Most scientists think that genetically engineering a virus which could infect humans is really very farfetched. Some would say that we do not, as yet, have the ability to be able to produce a genetically modified virus. However the conspiracy theory has found currency in some quarters. An ex-spymaster in the UK referred to a scientific paper that sections of the genetic sequence in Covid-19 had been inserted and that it is not a naturally occurring virus. This has led for claims from some quarters for China to pay reparations for the havoc it is created in the world.

But it is worth noting that the coronavirus is a marvellous and ingenious genetic machine. It is capable of mutating itself better than any human genetic engineer's attempts to change it!

It is interesting to note that Dr.Shi Zhengli stated that a future virus epidemic would originate in bats and that it was likely to start in China. Dr.Shi is a renowned virologist who has one of the largest world databases of bat –related viruses.

There is nothing wrong or immoral in collaborating with international colleagues in trying to understand issues that could be of global concern. The US ceased funding for experiments likely to produce dangerous germs because of fears of a pandemic, like the one the world is enduring at present.

The Chinese government refused to provide live viral samples to foreign scientists for analysis.

Huang Yan Ling was a researcher at the Wuhan Institute of Virology. There were rumours that she was the first to be diagnosed with Covid-19. She was therefore patient zero'. However she has disappeared and her details deleted from the website of the Institute.

Most of these viruses were found in bats in Guangdong province in China.

It is unlikely that the bats had flown several miles from their natural habitat to the city of Wuhan. It was likely that the virus was transferred there by either humans or other animals. Contrary to what was published it is unlikely that Chinese consumed 'bat soup' or ate bats. A researcher for the South China University of Technology, Xiaobo Tao" and also spelt as Botao Xiao, had published a report which stated that that researchers at 'Wuhan Virus Laboratory were splashed with bat blood and urine, and then quarantined for 14 days.' It was reported that bat were dissected and sometimes researchers were contaminated with urine and blood from the animals. It is known that bat urine and blood carry viruses.

It is therefore almost conclusive that Covid-19 originated in China. It is also possible that personnel working in the laboratory in Wuhan were infected with Covid-19, from where it spread to the local community. Tom Cotton a US Republican Senator said 'we don't know where it originated and we have to get to the bottom of that. We also know that just a few miles away from that food market is China's only bio-safety level four super-laboratory that researches human infectious diseases.' Another US official said that the Chinese may not have had any sinister intent but that they may have 'screwed up'.

Initially China attempted to blame the US for bringing the virus into Wuhan. The World Military Games were held in Wuhan in October 2019 and US athletes had travelled there. The Chinese claimed ' the US Army brought the epidemic to Wuhan. The Chinese Foreign Ministry wrote 'Be transparent! Make public your data! US owe us an explanation! As the story of the coronavirus unfolded the Chinese have remained silent on this allegation which has not been repeated.

Adding to the mystery about the origins of the virus and to all the conspiracy theories, there were reports that Dr. Shi Zhengli and her family had sought asylum in the United Sates embassy in Paris, taking several confidential documents with her. The rumour had no basis in fact as Dr. Shi Zhengli subsequently replied that defection 'shall never happen'.

Mathematical modelling by scientists in Southampton University in the UK suggests that if China had introduced lockdown three weeks earlier than it did, containment within China would have been more effective. This in turn would have reduced global spread. This view is accepted by some Chinese scientists too. Effective isolation and quarantine appeared to have helped limit the impact of SARS in 2003.

It was known around mid November 2019 that patients were being admitted to hospital in China with pneumonia. It is possible that a 55 year old man was the first person with Covid-19 – the 'Patient Zero'. Matthew Tye, a journalist, wrote that a researcher at the Wuhan Institute of Virology,

Huang Yanling, was patient zero. When a reporter from the Beijing News of the Mainland asked the WIV about the Huang Yanling it initially denied that she was a researcher at the Institute. But when WIV realised that such a person existed, it acknowledged that she had worked there but had since left and there was no record of her. Matthew Tye writes "Most people believe her to be patient zero, and most people believe she is dead'.

On 6th December 2019 five days after a man connected to Wuhan seafood market developed pneumonia, his wife contracted it. This suggests human to human transmission of the virus.

On 10th December 2019 another patient was admitted to hospital. He had worked in the seafood market in Wuhan. By 15th December there were 27 cases of the illness.

On 18th December 2019 a 65 year old man from Huanan market was admitted to hospital. Samples taken from his lung were sent for investigation on 24th December 2019. These showed that the fluid in his lung had coronavirus similar to the SARS virus of 2003. This patient subsequently died.

Samples from other patients who had been admitted also tested positive for the coronavirus.

On 27th December a researcher in a private firm in Guangzhou said the laboratory 'assembled a nearly complete viral genome sequence'. This information was obtained as part of an investigation by Caixin, an independent media group. The genomic sequence was passed by the laboratory to the Chinese Academy of Medical Sciences.

Another laboratory testing a Wuhan patient's sample completed the genomic sequence on 29th December 2019. Why was this information not shared with the WHO and the rest of the world at this stage? The WHO was aware that China was failing to share data. Had this information been available it may have helped contain the pandemic and prevent many unnecessary deaths.

On 30th December 2019 Dr. Li Wenliang who worked as an ophthalmologist (eye doctor) in Wuhan hospital shared, with colleagues on WeChat, information about patients with a SARS like infection in the hospital. WeChat is a Chinese internet social medium.

On this same day Dr. Shi Zhengli, virologist, was called to the Wuhan Institute of virology to help investigate the virus.

On 31ˢᵗ December 2019, China informed the WHO about the possibility of a new respiratory virus infection in Wuhan. It also informed the WHO that at that stage there was no evidence of human-to-human transmission.

On this date also the Chinese authorities began a crackdown on the spread of information about the infection. This is an important event, because it shows the extent to which China was prepared to suppress information exchange among its citizens. In doing so it also sought to prevent important information leaving the confines of China. This is unusual for us to experience in the UK; information is shared on the internet through email, Facebook etc. The Central Cyberspace Affairs Commission of China began censoring social media communications and discussion on the topic of an unknown infection. Apparently it removed references to Wuhan Market, pneumonia and several other bits of information. Similar action was taken in the Chinese YY streaming platform. Any reference to Dr. Wi Lenwiang, speculation, rumours etc. were deleted. This was an example of severe censoring of free speech from the outset. Researchers have found evidence of hundreds of Chinese people being fined or imprisoned for 'breaking Chinese Communist Party talking points'. One warning stated 'The police will investigate and deal with illegal acts of fabricating, disseminating, spreading rumours, and disturbing social order,'; 'It is hoped that the majority of citizens will abide by relevant laws and regulations, do not create rumours, believe rumours, or spread rumours, and jointly build a harmonious and clear cyberspace'.

It is vital to appreciate the impact of this aspect of the time line in the development of the global pandemic. Research from the University of Southampton showed that by their estimates there were 114,325 cases of Covid -19 in China by the end of February 2020. Their estimates showed that without intervention the number of cases would have been 67 times greater than what happened. The interventions available were early detection of cases, isolation and restriction on travel. Importantly the research showed that if these so called non –pharmaceutical intervention (NPI) had been done one, two and three weeks earlier the number of cases would have reduced by 66%, 86% and 95 percent respectively. But if the NPI's were done one, two and three weeks later than they were, the numbers of cases would have risen 3-fold, 7-fold and 18-fold respectively.

The authors also conclude social distancing and cancellation of large public events are important aspects in control of the disease.

In the early hours of 31 December 2019, Luo Yi-jun, deputy director for Taiwan's Centers for Disease Control, read on a public bulletin board, about an unknown disease causing pneumonia in Wuhan. He immediately placed Taiwan on alert.

On 1st January 2020 Wuhan food market was closed and disinfected. There is no way of knowing which animals, if any, carried the virus. All genomics companies were ordered by Hubei Health Commission to destroy all samples and to stop testing for the new virus. This had the effect of obliterating early information about the virus.

On 2nd January the Global Times of China tweeted - "Police in Central China's Wuhan arrested 8 people spreading rumours about local outbreak of unidentifiable pneumonia". This was censorship designed to silence people and prevent any discussion about the topic.

Vital early information was 'lost' and not shared with the WHO and the world.

On January 2nd Dr. Shi's team identified the genetic sequence of the virus. This showed that there was a link between the virus and horseshoe bats in Wuhan.

On January 3rd 2020 hospitals in China were ordered not to publish any details of cases of pneumonia or deaths. Also all samples taken from patients had to be sent to designated laboratories and apparently not tested in their own local laboratories. This may have been because the authorities wished to centralise testing in sites with sufficient skills or for another reason.

Also on 3rd January Dr. Li Wienlang, the initial whistleblower, was made by the police to sign a retraction of 'untruthful statements'.

On 4th January 2020 WHO used social media to inform that there was a cluster of patients with pneumonia in Wuhan.

On January 5th 2020 the genetic sequence of the virus was completed and it was identified as a respiratory virus.

On 5th January 2020 WHO informed the public and scientific community about what it had been told by China, about the presence of cases of pneumonia.

On January 9th 2019 the Mayor of Wuhan delivered his annual report to the local Communist Party Congress and failed to mention about the developing epidemic in the city. On this day or on the 10th of January the first death from the infection was recorded; a 61 year old man who shopped regularly at the Wuhan Seafood market. His wife also developed symptoms although she is not known to have visited the market. This makes it likely that transmission to her had occurred from him. But China maintained its stance that there is no human- to – human transmission of the virus and therefore, by inference, no transmission of the infection in the community.

Prof. Zhang Yongzhen of Shanghai placed the viral sequence in the public domain on 10th January.

On 12th January 2020 China published the genetic sequence of Covid-19. The WHO tweeted that it was 'reassured of the quality of the investigations and the response measures implemented on the novel coronavirus in Wuhan and the authorities commitment to share information with the WHO'. Prof. Yongzhen's laboratory was closed down for 'rectification'.

From the time line of events we know that there was secrecy and no desire by China to share information with its own citizens. Each delayed, controlled release of information contributed to global spread of the virus.

On 13th January a case of Covid-19 was identified in Thailand.; this was the first case outside of China.

On 14th January 2020 WHO informed the world that there was limited human-to-human transmission of the virus, mainly through family members. However it also tweeted 'preliminary investigations by the Chinese authorities have found no clear human-to – human transmission of the coronavirus'. But WHO knew of the man who died on 9th January and about the infection in his wife. If the WHO did not have this information, it was incumbent on them to have asked relevant questions in view of their experience with the paucity of information from China during the SARS epidemic. The WHO is clearly not an 'organisation with a memory'.

Around this time it was known that internal Communist Party documents reveal China's leaders knew that the country was facing an epidemic of the infection. On January 14th, Ma Xiaowei, who was a senior health official informed communist party colleagues about the situation.

In January there was a community gathering and banquet in Wuhan attended by about 50,000 families.

On January 20th the National Health Commission of China confirmed human-to human transmission of the virus. President Xi informed the Chinese public of the highly infectious nature of the disease.

On 22nd January 2020 the WHO China office informed that there was evidence of human-to –human transmission of the virus.

On 20th January 2020 a chest doctor publicly stated that the virus could be transmitted from person to person.

On 21st January the first case of Covid-19 was seen in Taiwan in a 50 year old female who had been teaching in Wuhan.

Lockdown was introduced in Wuhan on 23rd January 2020. WHO also reported that human-to-human transmission is possible with Covid-19. The Chinese authorities still warned its public not to spread rumours.

January 24th- authorities in China prevent Wuhan Institute of Virology from sharing samples with the University of Texas.

Chinese New Year was on 25th January and it is likely that millions of people would have been travelling home, visiting families and friends etc. Considering this mass movement of people it is surprising that the numbers infected by and who died from Covid-19 in China were small. About five million people are known to have left Wuhan, carrying the virus far and wide.

On 26th January 2020 Taiwan suspended all flights between it and China.

On January 30th 2020 the Director General of the WHO, Tedros Adhnom Ghebreyesus, praised China in a tweet "setting a new standard for outbreak response'. Considering the timeline of events this was either a gross understatement or worse still, delusional. The WHO was aware that China was holding back releasing vital information about the virus. Importantly China was aware of human-to-human transmission of the virus but did not share this information before 20th January. Under international law countries are obliged to inform the WHO on matter that could have an adverse impact on public health. But it cannot enforce this. The WHO has to rely on cooperation from countries.

April 17th - Mortality from Covid-19 in Wuhan is belatedly raised to 1290.

Dr. Mike Ryan, executive director of WHO's health emergencies program said that WHO was reassured that the virus was natural in origin.

Dr. Li Wenliang who first raised concerns about Covid 19 on 30th December 2019 died himself of Covid-19 on 7th February 2020. He was 33 years old. The Times newspaper in the UK reported his death and wrote that his early whistle-blowing was 'a case study in Beijing's kneejerk suppression and control of information'. When the Chinese public heard about his death there was great sadness. The response from the authorities was to cynically claim 'that he was critically ill and being resuscitated'. There could surely be very few more disgusting responses to the death of another being than this one. And a blatant lie from the rulers of China.

About the middle of March 2020 a message from China said: 'An inspection team of the National Supervisory Commission released the report of an investigation into issues related to Dr. Li Wenliang, an ophthalmologist with the Central Hospital of Wuhan. Following the report, Wuhan Public Security Bureau decided to revoke the previous reprimand letter and apologized to Li's family over the mistake.'

Dr. Li and fourteen other medical personnel who worked in Hubei and died from Covid-19 have received the title of 'martyr. All were mourned on National Mourning Day for victims of Covid-19. Dr. Li was 'lauded for his bravery, dedication and quick reaction'. A Chinese Central TV post said: 'they disregarded their personal safety, stuck to the front line, raced against the clock fighting the demon illness and safeguard people's life safety and health day and night'.

Subsequently it was revealed that Dr. Li Wenliang acted after receiving a text message from a colleague, Dr. Ai Fen. Dr Ai worked in the emergency department and criticised Wuhan Central Hospital for dismissing early warnings of the coronavirus. Following the death of Dr. Li, she expressed regret for not being more vocal about her concerns about the virus. As expected Dr. Ai was detained and it is reported that she has not been seen since she gave an interview on 10th March to Renwu, a Chinese magazine. It is said that Dr. Ai Fen is 'the one who gave out the whistles to the whistle-blowers'.

Interesting information has been presented relating to hospital activity in the months prior to China declaring to the WHO about Covid-19. Researchers from Harvard Medical School used satellite imagery to look at how busy hospital car parks were in Wuhan in 2019 compared to the same period in 2018. The research team looked at 111 satellite images. Some of the images were not useful for comparison because of cloud cover. In Zhongnan University Hospital, Wuhan there were 506 cars parked on a day in October 2018 but 640 cars parked on a day in October 2019. In Tongji Medical University in Wuhan the number of cars parked was 112 on one day in October 2018 compared to 214 on a day in September 2019. And finally in Wuhan Tianyou Hospital there were 171 car parked on a day in October 2018 compared to 285 in 2019. The vehicular traffic appeared to have reached its peak in mid-December 2019. Around the same time there was a marked rise in the use of the Chinese internet search engine, Baidu. Users were looking up the terms 'cough' and 'diarrhoea'. The conclusion of the researchers was that while this information constitutes circumstantial evidence, it still points to some kind of 'social disruption' taking place in the Wuhan area at the time. The paper by the researchers has not been peer reviewed. Critics have expressed concern that some of the hospitals reviewed in the images were children's hospitals. Children are not known to suffer in large numbers from Covid-19. Others say that children's hospitals may be been requisitioned for adult use if there were significant numbers of patients.

Several athletes who attended the Military World Games in Wuhan in October 2019 fell ill. These included Spanish, French and German sportsmen and sports women. In one instance all six occupants in an official apartment of the games fell ill. There is no evidence that any of these athletes subsequently tested positive for Covid -19. While the information is again circumstantial there is no clear evidence that all the sport people who fell ill in Wuhan did so form Covid-19.

Researchers at the Albert Schweitzer Hospital in north-eastern France reviewed all chest scans done between 1st November 2019 and 30th April 2020. There were about 2500 scans looked at. They identified two scans done in mid- November 2019 which they say is 'consistent 'with Covid-19. 'The first case was noted in our centre on November 16th 'said Dr.Michel Schmitt, the chief radiologist of the hospital.

A Hong Kong newspaper, The South China Morning Post, reported that the first case of Covid-19 can be traced back to 17th November 2019.

There are three strains of the virus. Virus type A is that found in bats in the caves in China and was found in patients in Australia and the USA. Virus type B was found in patients in China and Type C in patients in Europe.

China was accused of deliberately suppressing or destroying evidence of the virus outbreak in an "assault on international transparency". The effect of this was the death of thousands of people across the world. It was able to do this by silencing people within China, some of whom have disappeared.

Sir John Sawer, a former head of MI6 in the UK, accused China of concealing information for two months. He also indicated that the WHO had 'serious questions' to answer as to why it did not hold China to account. The WHO had not asked the right questions and appeared to have accepted what was said by China. The delay of six days prior to the announcement by President Xi Jinping on 20th January contributed to deaths not only in Wuhan but allowed spread of the virus and additional avoidable deaths.

On March 2020 the official Chinese news agency, Xinhua, claimed that the world should thank China for its sacrifices in dealing with the infection and thereby allowing the rest of the world to obtain a valuable window of time to prepare for the pandemic. It is timely to ask what these sacrifices were. If at all, the people of Wuhan were lambs to the slaughter. When the alarm was raised by Dr. Li, and given China's previous experience with SARS, it should have acted quickly in containing the infection. On the contrary the authorities consigned the population of Wuhan and far afield to the risk of infection and death.

The Mayor of Wuhan, Zhou Xianwang, tendered his resignation because information was not released as early as it should have been.

A study has found that if China acted three weeks earlier, than it did, in alerting the world medical community, the number of cases worldwide could have reduced by 95%

It is understood that over 5000 people in China were arrested for spreading information about the outbreak of Covid-19.

Should the world believe what China says? When one uses the word "China' one is actually referring to the Chinese Communist Party (CCP). The CCP controls all life and activities in China. It is a totalitarian regime which exerts influence on and control of life in China and some would even say beyond its borders. Some writers refer to 'grotesque deceptions' by the CCP in relation to Covid-19.

Prior to the recent virus infection it is known that a strain of flu appeared din 1977 in China and parts of Russia and spread around the world. It mainly affected young persons. It was a H1N1 strain of influenza virus that had first appeared in the mid 1950's. The virus had apparently remained dormant. There was thought to have been an accidental release of the frozen dormant virus that was held in a laboratory in China. It was called Russian flu. How the virus remained dormant for over 20 years has not been explained. The possibility of concealed experimentation has not been excluded. The relevance of this event is important in the light of Covid-19. Could experimentation have again led to the escape of the coronavirus from a laboratory in China?

Information regarding bio-security in its laboratories and about the occurrence of infections in people was controlled following the onset of Covid-19. This is a common response by the CCP and helps it to control the narrative and to portray China in the best light. The eventual story that emerges may have little bearing on what actually happened or continued to happen after the event. The CCP continually lies to its people. Take the train crash of 2011. On 23rd July 2011 two high speed trains collided in Wnezhou killing forty people and injured almost 200 others. The accident happened on a viaduct, off which four of the cars fell. The response of the Chinese authorities was the immediate burial of the derailed cars and strict media censorship about the event. The cause of the accident was poor engineering design followed by incompetent subsequent management.

On 12th May 2008 an earthquake of magnitude 7.8 on the Richter scale occurred in Sichuan. This was a devastating earthquake with tremors felt in Taiwan, Mongolia, Russia, India, Bangladesh, Pakistan and Thailand. About 69,000 people died in Sichuan and 375,000 were injured. The Tzu Chi Foundation from Taiwan was the first country from outside of China to respond on 13th May. China appealed for international help to deal with the catastrophe. Other countries that stepped in with help were South Korea, Russia, USA, Japan and Singapore. The United Nations International Children's Emergency Fund (UNICEF) appealed for international help to support affected Chinese families and children.

Following the earthquake Chinese media openly reported events, prompting one Peking University professor to state - "This is the first time the Chinese media has lived up to international standards". In a similar vein the Los Angeles Times praised Chinese media for being democratic in providing information about the earthquake.

However, initial Chinese reports for over a week following the earthquake were of only a few fatalities. Chinese authorities also prevented people from protesting, often offering bribes of money to encourage people to remain silent. Many refused to do so. In one province, parents who had lost children were offered US$ 8000 and a pension for each parent of US$ 5,600. Riot police were used to break up crowds and people and the media were prevented from coming near to or reporting about collapsed schools. Liu Shaokun, a school teacher, had taken photographs of collapsed school buildings and posted them online. He was arrested on 25th June and investigated on the suspicion of inciting subversion. He was sentenced to one year of 're-education through labour' (RTL). These events are reminiscent of the fate of the whistleblower, Dr. Li Wenliang, aged 34 years, who first raised awareness of Covid-19. RTL reminds one of what is currently happening to the Uighurs in China.

The Covid-19 epidemic brought its share of prisoners in China. Mr. Fang Bin is a Chinese businessman and whistleblower. He posted several pictures of Wuhan on YouTube and WeChat, the Chinese platform. His first video was on 25th January 2020. On the 1st February 2020 he posted a video of corpses being piled into a van in front of Wuhan hospital. A picture also showed body bags piled outside the hospital. He was arrested and warned not to spread rumours. He released his last video On February 9 with the words "resist all citizens, hand the power of the government back to the people". He was arrested and has not been seen since.

Dr. Li Wenliang's lawyer, Chen Qiushi and a former state TV reporter Li Zehua were also arrested and have not appeared. They have been euphemistically 'disappeared'. This is likely to have been incarceration and torture until they confess to their crimes. They were considered enemies of the state. It is known that in excess of 5000 people were arrested for sharing information at the outset of the infection in China. Interestingly dissidents were labelled as being 'sick' and placed in medical quarantine.

Li Zehua's case is interesting. Aged 25 years he was a reporter with Chinese state TV. He not only had the courage to tell the public on TV about the death toll in Wuhan but also published his own arrest when police officers visited his flat.

There is no information about these three people.

The billionaire property developer and Communist Party member Ren Zhiqiang was an outspoken critic of the government. In a message he called the Chinese leader, Xi Jinping, a clown for the manner in which the coronavirus outbreak was handled. He too was arrested in March and has not been seen since then. Similar punishment was meted to law professor, Xu Zhangrun, for criticising Xi Jinping.

The disappearance and silencing of dissenters and those who act against the CCP is a means of frightening the population into submission. True to an old Chinese idiom, the authorities would 'kill a chicken to frighten the monkey'. It is a way of making an example of a few so as to threaten and subdue the majority. These are examples of extreme control, worse than any form authoritarianism. This is control of speech and of thought and any of form of 'adverse 'communication with others. The only permitted voice of the Chinese and the only narrative that is allowed is that which emanates from the CCP. This is important for the CCP's command and control system of government. It is designed to avoid mass dissatisfaction among its population, which could easily lead to widespread revolt, as has happened in the past.

The Chinese people deserve the world's wholesome plaudits and bouquets. And to the Chinese Communist Party are reserved nothing but brickbats. The former have a right to better. The CCP have only humiliated the country and its proud people.

Who is Dr. Tedros Adhanom Ghebreyesus, the current Director-General of the WHO? It is useful to understand his role in the Covid-19 crisis that has enveloped the entire globe. Dr.Tedros Adhanom Ghebreyesus, also known as Dr. Tedros, was born on 3rd of March 1965 in Asmara in the original Ethiopia. Asmara is now in Eritrea. Ethiopia was the second most populous state in Africa after Nigeria, before it split into two separate countries, Ethiopia and Eritrea following a long civil war that ran from 1961 to 1991. Ethiopia was ruled by Emperor Haile Selasse. The emperor was deposed in 1974 by a military junta called Derg, made up of lower ranking army officers, police and the territorial army. It was also called the Coordinating Committee of the Armed Forces, Police and Territorial

Army which eventually changed its name to the Provisional Military Administrative Council. The DERG was communist and abolished the monarchy of Emperor Haile Selasse. Thereafter the country was run as a one- parry Marxist state. Mengistu Haile Mariam became President in 1977. He proceeded to eliminate political opponents by imprisonment, torture and execution without trial.

After 1977 Derg was in war with rebels from Tigray and the Tigrayan Peoples' Liberation Front. To enable it in its battles with opponents Ethiopia received aid from Russia which was then the Union of Soviet Socialist republics (USSR), North Korea and East Germany. The constant wars led to reduced economic activity and reduced productivity. This led to the famine of 1980 which was made worse by drought. In 1991 a coalition of rebels forces called the Ethiopian People's Revolutionary Democratic Front (EPRDF) eventually forced Mengistu out and he sought asylum in Zimbabwe.

Dr.Tedros, as I shall call him, graduated in biology from the University of Asmara in Eritrea in 1986. At the age of 23 he spent a few months studying in Denmark. He did a master's degree in the immunology of infectious disease at the London School of Hygiene and Tropical Medicine in 1992. He also studied at the University of Nottingham where he received a PhD in community medicine in 2000. He does not a have a primary degree in medicine and is the first Director General of the WHO in its entire 72 history who is not a medical doctor.

After graduation from Asmara, Dr.Tedros worked as a health official in the government of President Mengistu Haile Mariam. He then joined the Tigray Peoples Liberation Front. This was a communist party and contributed to President Mengistu being deposed and seeking exile. TPRF became a powerful armed rebel group in Ethiopia. Dr. Tedros was claimed to be one for the top three people in the TPLF which is said to be responsible for kidnapping, mass detention and torture of civilians. It was also involved in forceful acquisition of lands and of causing displacement of people. Tigray is one of nine regional states comprising Ethiopia which at the time was run as a federation. Tigray was also known as Region 1. The regions or federations were based on ethno-linguistic groups and hence could be seen as having been racial in their separation of people. Tigray is populated by Tigrayans. Tigrayans, however, comprise only

6% of the population of Ethiopia. The two larger ethnic groups, the Oromo (34%) and Amharic (30%) are effectively marginalised, with many having migrated and comprising a significant diaspora. Senior posts in the military, in other parts of the security system and in several state institutions are occupied by Tigrayans.

The USA classed the TPLF as a terrorist organisation.

Dr.Tedros held various posts in health in Ethiopia. In 2001 he was head of the Tigray Regional Health Bureau followed by deputy minister of health in Ethiopia in 2003 and minister of health in 2005. He was involved in national and global health activities like controlling malaria, HIV/AIDS, family planning etc. While Dr. Tedros was health minister the occurrence of HIV/AIDS, which was one of the highest in Ethiopia, was significantly reduced.

He became minister of foreign affairs in 2012, which post he held until 2016. Critics of Dr. Tedros say that he was complicit in the arbitrary arrest, detention and torture of people who were opposed to the government. The government of the time was repressive and imposed extremely tough censorship laws which some say were the most severe in the world at the time.

The strongest opposition to the election of Dr. Tedros to the post of Director-General of WHO came from Ethiopians. Human Rights Watch found that donor money given for basic services was used to promote teachers and farmers to join the ruling party although this was forbidden in the donor program. It was also said that money was used to help opposition members to write to the party asking for 'forgiveness' so that they had access to food.

There was evidence of bribery, cronyism and discrimination in the way food, for example, was distributed.

What is particularly worrying is that during the election to the post of Director General information came to light that Dr. Tedros had concealed three epidemics of cholera in Ethiopia during his tenure as minister of health in the country. Lawrence Gostin, a lawyer, is also Professor of Public Health at the Johns Hopkins University and Georgetown University. The latter is a Collaborating Centre of the World Health Organization. He is also a Professor of Public Health at Oxford University. He was an advisor to Dr.David Nabarro at the time the latter was in contention with

Dr.Tedros for the post of Director-General. Lawrence Gostin highlighted the cover-up by Ethiopia of its cholera epidemics, while stating in the New York Times newspaper that the WHO "might lose its legitimacy" if it is run by someone who failed to "speak truth to power," and who had covered up epidemics.

There were epidemics of cholera in Ethiopia in 2006, 2009 and in 2011, but these were not recorded as such. According to the New York Times these cases were recorded as "acute watery diarrhoea,". Now diarrhoea is one of the cardinal symptoms of cholera. Subsequently international investigators looked at stool samples from patients and identified Vibrio cholerae, the bacterium that is the cause of cholera. This was an example of institutionalised concealment of diagnosis which at its worst does not permit effective management of patients and the prevention of transmission of an infectious disease to other persons.

Dr.Tedors was elected in a secret ballot of three rounds with six candidates vying for the post of Director General. He eventually won against the two final contenders, Dr. Sania Nishtar, of Pakistan, and Dr. David Nabarro, of Britain. Most if not all African nations voted for Dr.Tedros, who is the first Africa to occupy the post of Director General.

Co-Director of the Health Observatory at the Institute of International Relations (IRIS), Anne Sénéquier says "Tedros thinks like a politician, not like a doctor." This is an important observation and may go some way to explain his conduct during the early stages of the coronavirus pandemic.He did not appreciate or he set aside the medical risks of what was evolving. Instead he appeared to proceed as a politician and as a diplomat. He attempted to maintain dialogue with the Chinese authorities and accepted their explanations without challenge. She does not doubt that he contributed much as a heath minster in Ethiopia. But she also maintains that "He has built hospitals and medical schools; he has done a lot in terms of volume, but not in terms of quality. Everything was underfunded, and for many, this infrastructural push was more political than clinical in the sense that it did not improve the quality of the health care system. And like a politician, the more you attack him, the more he resists".

'There are none so blind as those who will not see'!

China is a big investor in Ethiopia. China sees Ethiopia as an important partner in its Belt and Road Initiative (BRI). The BRI is a long-term project by China to establish its ancient trading routes toward the Suez Canal and then onwards Europe.

All the previous Directors-General of the WHO had been medically qualified. Dr. Tedros' predecessor was Dr.Margaret Chan, a Chinese-Canadian doctor who qualified in medicine from the University of Western Ontario in Canada. She had served as Director of Health in Hong Kong and managed the outbreaks of avian influenza in 1997 and of severe acute respiratory syndrome (SARS) in 2003. Dr Chan was elected as Director-General of WHO on 9 November 2006 and followed this by being re-appointed to the post for a second term, which ended on 30 June 2017. Her management of the SARS outbreak was much criticised by the public in Hong Kong where 299 people died. Subsequently an investigation by the Hong Kong government exonerated her and said that death were due to faults in the way the health care system worked.

During a visit to North Korea in 2010 she commented that obesity was not a problem in that country although her predecessor as Director General of WHO said in 2001 that the country's health care system was near collapse. The Wall Street Journal implied in its comments that Dr.Chan was ignoring reality.

The difficulty the WHO has in dealing with epidemics is seen in the way Dr.Chan was accused in some quarters of over-reacting to the 2009 flu epidemic. Epidemics and pandemic, by their nature, are rapidly changing situations and it is not possible to be precise in advising how they should be dealt with.

Gordon Chang of Fox News said that "Tedros is the second-to-last person who should be heading the World Health Organization at this time; the last person is (Chinese President) Xi Jinping."

Early on in the pandemic Dr. Tedros tweeted "For the first time, China has reported no domestic COVID19 cases yesterday. This is an amazing achievement, which gives us all reassurance that the coronavirus can be beaten,". This is a premature statement considering the recurrence of Covid-19 in Beijing in June 2020.

o0:0o

ANATOMY OF A DISASTER

'No definite grounds. But the symptoms are definitely alarming'

'The figures are going up, doctor. Eleven deaths in forty-eight hours'

'if the epidemic did not cease spontaneously, it would be necessary to apply rigorous prophylactic measures'

"I know. The figures are rising."

'putting into force some precautionary measures'

'he had to undergo a spell of quarantine'

'a desire not to alarm the public'

'persons living in the same house were to go into quarantine'

'Hostile to the past, impatient of the present, and cheated of the future, we were much like *prisoners*'

'The mortality figures....... showed a decrease'

'the *virus* never dies or disappears for good; it can lie dormant for years and years …and perhaps the day would come when …it would *rise up again*'

These are statements which the reader may be familiar with, since Covid-19 hit the UK. Some may even claim to recognise them, having heard them on TV or read them in newspapers during the current pandemic.

But these words are taken from the book, The Plague, by Albert Camus which was published in 1948. We see some of the scenes in the book being played out in our daily lives, in our communities and in the country as a whole.

On 12th March 2020, Boris Johnson, Prime Minister of UK, said 'More families, many more families are going to lose loved ones before their time.'

How did we come to this? Given the exponential human progress of the past seventy years, it is sometimes difficult to imagine how we are here.

It has been recognised for some time that there are few events more catastrophic to society than to be affected by a lethal epidemic. One of the oldest known epidemics wiped out an entire village in China about 5000 years ago. Children, young adults and older people died. Dead bodies were stuffed inside a house which was subsequently burned down. It is now a well preserved archaeological site called 'Hamin Mangha' in north-eastern China. A similar mass burial site was found in Miaozigou in the same region of China. Plagues have occurred since then leading to deaths of large numbers of people.

In January 2020 scientific advisors in the UK knew that the Covid-19 virus had the same potential to spread and infect people as the virus of the Spanish flu in 1918. In that epidemic almost a quarter of the world's population was infected and up to 100 million people died from it.

On 17th January there were the first reports of two cases of the virus infection outside China, one in Thailand and the second in Japan. This is serious, for now the virus had crossed national boundaries and confirmed the possibility of human-to human transmission of the virus. How many people in China and elsewhere were infected with the virus was not known, as not everyone infected with the virus would have had symptoms. But everyone with the virus would spread it to others and there was the potential that the infection could spread like a wild fire across the country. This should have been an alert to anyone concerned with the spread of viral influenza and chest infections. To the UK government's NERVTAG (New And Emerging Respiratory Virus Threat Advisory Group) this information should have been like a red rag to a bull. There should have been heightened concern about spread to the UK and also about the vulnerability of large segments of the population to Covid-19, as it was later to be called.

In late February 2020 scientific advisors warned the government that in excess of 250,000 people could die of the virus unless preventive measures were taken and effective lockdown was implemented. The figure of 250,000 was arrived at from what was known about the virus, previous experience of viruses like SARS, avian flu etc and mathematical modelling of risk to the public. Modelling is not an exact science – it is a best estimate of what could happen, based on the available evidence at the time. The figure of 250,000 deaths would have had a range extending from a lower figure to one which would have been much higher. This is the best that modelling could provide and the range tells us how confident the scientists are with the estimate. Of course the number can change with changing circumstances and evidence. Covid-19 is a moving target and evidence of risk of infection and spread was changing all the time. These do not make the science bad, only that the figure of 250,000 deaths is the best result from the calculations of the time. Many factors are taken into account in a modelling exercise and any one or more of these could affect the results that are obtained. But, and to recount the words of the late Margaret Thatcher, ex-Prime Minister, there is no alternative (TINA). Modelling is a necessity to help appreciate how an event like the pandemic would affect the country. Take the example of deaths on roads. Modelling of available information on deaths and various types of interventions to reduce deaths, for e.g. road signs, one-way systems, speed restrictions etc would give a best estimate of the most effective action to reduce accidents and deaths on a particular stretch of road. But whatever is done, it is never possible to eliminate all accidents and deaths.

As at 3rd March 2020 there were 51 cases of Covid-19 in England and the NHS Chief Medical Officer, Chris Witty, said that at the extreme it was possible 80% of the population would be infected, with most getting a mild disease. He also suggested that 1% of patients would die and this would affect the elderly more than the young. By this estimate 500,000 people would die from the infection.

The advice to government at the time was that lockdown would limit spread of the virus in the community (lower R number) and help reduce the rate of infection.

China notified the WHO on 31st December 2019 that there were several cases of an unusual pneumonia in Wuhan.

The government's Scientific Advisory Group for Emergencies (SAGE) met on 22nd January when it was recognised that the virus had an infectivity rate of 3. This is called the R figure or reproduction number, and in this instance was R3. There are 3 possible values for R – R of less than one means that each infected person is likely to spread the virus to less than one person causing a new case of infection. So an R of 0.5 would mean that two people with the virus are likely to spread and cause only one new case. R of 1 means that each case would cause another new case i.e. reproduce a new case of the virus infection. R greater than 1 means that each case would cause the corresponding number of new cases. So R of 3 means one person could spread the infection to three other persons.

As Paolo Giordano explains to us in his book, 'How Contagion Works', R is not something picked out of the air. Imagine a seed planted in soil grows and produces three branches. Imagine now that each one of those branches also grows to produce 3 of its own branches and each of the new branches does the same. Now let's say that each new branch that continues to appear on the tree does the same producing 3 branches. Soon we would end with a vast bushy tree; like a vast spreading oak tree. If, on the other hand, the seed produced only a single stalk of the plant without spreading branches, there would have been a slender tree. Giordano helps us understand that the first seed that produced three branches and so on has a R value of 3 while the second seed has a R of zero as it did not produce any branches at all. So an infection with the chance of infecting two others and so on could have a disastrous effect on the spread of the infection. Very soon large sections of the community would be infected and finally a vast number of people in the entire country would be infected. Some of those infected would not have any symptoms but still contribute to the R figure by spreading the infection to others. Some would die from the infection - which gave rise to the mathematical estimate of 250,000 deaths from Covid-19. The aim of infection control is to keep R as far below 1 as possible, when the risk of spread and the appearance of new cases of the infection would be quite limited.

Measles for e.g. has an R of 12-18. This means that in the absence of vaccination it would spread rapidly and infect many people. The UK was able to eliminate measles based on information from 2014-2016. But the UK lost this status of elimination in 2018 because there were 284 cases of measles in 2017 and 991 cases in England and Wales in 2018. As a result of these figures showing re-emergence of measles, the WHO removed the measles elimination status from the UK in 2018. In comparison, worldwide, there were about 10 million cases of measles in 2018 with 142,000 deaths. In the first three months of 2019 there were 83,540 cases of measles in the European region with 53,218 of these in Ukraine alone. With a R number of 12-18 for measles and one thousand cases of measles as the UK had in 2018, there would have been a severe epidemic of measles in England if most of the population had not been vaccinated against measles virus.

Smallpox, another deadly viral infection, on the other hand has a R of 3-6. But because it is eliminated, immunity in public (herd immunity) is low. Therefore, if small-pox were to reappear, many of us would become infected very quickly. In the 18th century small-pox used to kill more than 10% of the British population. Then a successful vaccine was developed by Edward Jenner from cow pox. Cowpox is also called Vaccinia, which lends its name to vaccines and vaccination. Small pox has been eliminated worldwide and is lasting proof of how effective vaccination is in controlling the spread of some infections. Those who are opposed to vaccination have chosen to ignore the lessons of history. The work of Jenner has vital resonance today as scientists around the world work to develop a vaccine that could contain and hopefully eliminate Covid-19.

In the case of the Spanish flu epidemic of 1918 the R figure was 1.4 to 2.8 and the flu caused nearly 100 million deaths. It was caused by the H1N1 virus. When the same H1N1 swine flu virus came back in 2009 the R value was 1.4 to 1.6 resulting in a far less number of cases and deaths. Of course the improvements in personal and public health and in medicine in the intervening years have helped to limit spread of infection and to reduce people's susceptibility to it.

In 2020 therefore, it was imperative that action was taken soon to stop the spread of the coronavirus. This would have required an immediate lockdown. However such a drastic step did not seem to be acceptable to the government at the time.

Cabinet Office Briefing Rooms (COBR) are a series of rooms in the Cabinet Office at 70 Whitehall, London where the Prime Minister of the day, members of the cabinet and others meet to discuss important issues. These may be national or regional crises or international matters where there may be implications for the UK. These meetings are called COBRA meetings despite there not being the letter A; it is a useful acronym. The

Prime Minister chairs these meetings which are attended by some cabinet ministers, and other relevant persons for e.g. the Police, military, local mayors etc.

At the COBRA meeting of 24th January the public were reassured that the situation was being monitored by experts and that there were no confirmed cases of the virus in the UK. This COBRA meeting lasted an hour before it was concluded that the risk to the UK was 'low'. On the same day the Lancet medical journal carried an article by doctors from China implying that the virus had the potential to spread. Downing Street maintained that the UK was 'well prepared for any new diseases'. However, this was seriously worrying complacency. It is uncertain if the concerns and fears of scientists were dismissed by politicians at this stage. Scientists had warned the government about the emerging threat from the virus and of the possibility of large numbers of dead. The Secretary for Health, Matt Hancock, said after the meeting 'the clinical advice is that the risk to the public remains low'. Professor Paul Cosford, emeritus medical director at PHE, said it is still 'early days' and followed up by saying 'I think it's highly likely that we will have cases in the UK.' At this stage the reported number of deaths in China was 26 with the number of confirmed cases of Covid-19 being 830.

In the whole of February the Prime Minister, Boris Johnson, did not attend any of the COBRA meetings that took place to discuss the emerging crisis. This was the time when there was a significant amount of flooding in parts of the country, with which the Prime Minister may have been pre-occupied. To have missed these meeting must weigh heavily and the impression created was of a government not in control and of failing to recognise the evolving danger to the public. As a result of this lapse, several weeks of planning and activity were lost since the publication in the Lancet medical journal on 24th January implying person-to person transmission of Covid-19.

At the time of the COBRA meeting of 24th January there was evidence of human-to-human transmission of the virus. WHO had stated in a press briefing on 14th January that there was the risk of a wider outbreak of the infection. It expected human-to-human transmission to occur, given evidence from the previous SARS and MERV epidemics.

On January 16th, alarmed by what was going on in Wuhan, Professor of Global Public Health from Edinburgh, Devi Sridhar, was on Twitter calling for immediate action to deal with the likelihood of the infection in the UK.

Professor Neil Ferguson and his team from Imperial College, London produced evidence from their first modelling on 17th January of the risks from the virus. The data showed that there was at that stage likely to have been about 4000 cases and the likelihood of human-to-human transmission of infection could not be ruled out. The report called for increased surveillance and preparedness.

January and February were months when the country was sleepwalking towards a catastrophe. The government had been advised about the possibility of 210,000 to 315,000 deaths in as short a period as 15 weeks from the onset of the pandemic in the UK. The virus was spreading through crowds at stations, in trains, at airports and workplaces etc. It was also spreading silently in care homes. These were five weeks that were lost in the battle against coronavirus and during which time the virus had gained the upper hand. Disaster was soon to engulf the country with a rising number of deaths.

On 22nd January the first meeting of the Scientific Advisory Group for Emergencies (SAGE) in the UK took place. It had information that the infectivity rate of the virus, that is the R figure, was 3. This meant that each person with the virus could in turn infect three other people, and the process of transmission of the infection could go on. With this likely rate of spread of the infection, lockdown was imperative to cut the rate of transmission of the infection to 60% or less. This could only be achieved by stopping people being in contact with each other. This in turn meant a shutdown of the economy, schools, recreation and virtually any activity involving human contact.

After the COBRA meeting of 25th January, the Chief Medical Office, Chris Whitty, said that the situation was being monitored by experts and that there were no confirmed cases of Covid-19 in the UK.

The UK government did not appear to have been proactive at this stage. During January and February 2020 there was no apparent action on the part of government to review emergency planning for a pandemic or to verify whether the available pandemic plan was fit for its current purpose. Most importantly there did not seem to have been any activity regarding reserves of equipment like ventilators and disposables like PPE, should they be needed at short notice. The country was poorly prepared for the pandemic.

January and February were crucial months when, even without and prior to lockdown there should have been active replenishment of stocks of necessary material to manage the pandemic. This must surely be the most significant failure of government and probably consigned the country to a greater epidemic and larger death rate from Covid-19 than would otherwise have been the case.

The NHS has a long history of managing the logistics and supply of various types of health care products to NHS institutions nationwide. The NHS Supply Chain was created in 2016 and in April 2018 the operation of NHS Supply Chain went to a limited company, Supply Chain Coordination Limited, which is wholly owned by the Secretary of State for Health and Social Care. One of the objectives of NHS Supply Chain is 'to leverage the buying power of the NHS to negotiate the best deals from supplier'. It is interesting to ask why the skills of NHS Supply Chain were not used at the outset to obtain all that was likely to be needed to manage the pandemic. It was also vital to ensure that supply chains remain viable and able to meet the continuing needs of the UK. We now know that with the global pandemic there were extraordinary strains on international supply chains, trying to meet demands from many countries. Being proactive may have helped the UK in containing the virus and in having adequate supplies to deal with infection.

The Department of Health was advised by an independent committee in 2019 to stockpile PPE. The National Audit Office (NAO) had reported that at the start of the pandemic the only central stock of PPE held by the Public Health England was designated for use in the pandemic. However it lacked gowns and visors. These items would be considered basic protection material to help combat an infection. That these were not available is an indictment of preparedness despite the availability of plans precisely for dealing with such a situation. Following a request from China for help, the government sent it 279,000 items of PPE from its own depleted stock. This added to shortages and to the risk that the UK eventually had to contend with.

Then, less than a week later, on 30th January 2020 the Director General of WHO informed the world that Covid-19 is a Public Health Emergency of International Concern (PHEIC). PHEIC is a critical notice to countries that a serious medical emergency is likely to develop. At this stage the numbers of cases worldwide had risen to 7818 with the majority of cases being in China. Eighty-two cases had been reported from 18 countries. The appearance of cases in other countries should have raised concerns that the UK was likely to be affected by the virus.

Covid-19 was first detected in the UK in two Chinese citizens on 29th January 2020. They were staying at the Staycity Aparthotel in York. These two cases were followed by a British businessman in Brighton. He caught the disease in Singapore. On February 28th a man in Surrey got the virus infection; he had not been abroad.

Covid-19 was now upon us and likely to increase exponentially, as it eventually did across many countries. So, as of the end of February the UK had Covid-19 cases in persons who had come from abroad. It is reasonable to assume they had contracted the virus abroad. How many people they had transmitted the virus to when in the UK is not known. The man from Brighton illustrates that the virus was now in the community and spreading.

The stage was now set for the UK to gather information from other countries about the virus, increase surveillance in the UK and consider testing for the virus.

On 6th February the 53 year old man from Brighton in Sussex was the second source of spread of the virus. But PHE failed to pursue a course of testing and tracing. Necessary equipment for testing was not ordered, which subsequently led to problems. The British in vitro Diagnostics Association claimed that it had not been approached by the government for help with testing equipment.

On 7th February the WHO Scientific and Technical Advisory Group for Infectious Hazards (STAG-IH) 'concluded that the continuing strategy of containment for elimination should continue, and that the coming 2–3 weeks through to the end of February 2020, will be crucial to monitor the situation of community transmission.' However, it is known that large numbers of travellers were still flying into Britain. Between January and March 2020, 18 million people flew into Britain. According to the University of Southampton 190,000 people flew into UK airports from

Wuhan and other parts of China. There is no doubt, many of these travellers had the virus, which they then proceeded to spread to communities in the UK. It was estimated that about 1900 of these travellers had the virus. This was the time the infection was spreading in UK. It was reported that at least 20,000 infected people arrived in the UK before lockdown was introduced. Australia banned foreign travellers arriving from China. Although the WHO had said that stopping flights 'was the worst thing one could do for a global health crisis' Professor Sharon Lewin, a public health specialist, said that doing so 'saved Australia, because it actually stopped seeding at the very beginning.' Without limiting flights into Britain and without quarantine of those who had arrived here, it was obvious that the pool of infection in the country was increasing. Also the spread of infection may have been increasing exponentially due to the R number of the time. Here surely was a medical 'bomb' waiting to explode!

On Friday 28th February there were 19 cases of Covid-19 in UK. It was also the day in which the London stock market plummeted. The FTSE index which was 7358 at the beginning of February closed at 6796 on 28th February, a drop of 8% causing £152 billion to be wiped off the value of stocks. At the time of this writing the index had dropped to 6032. The urgency of the situation was finally recognised.

The UK had the Pandemic Preparedness Plan which stated that it would not be possible to avoid an infection in the UK. Human-to-human transmission was known to occur and large numbers of people were still travelling into the UK. And the UK, even at the end of February, had not acted to curtail the spread of infection or to replenish PPE stocks.

At the COBRA meeting of March 2nd attended by the Prime Minister, the country moved into some action in creating the Nightingale Hospitals. But it was not until 23rd March that the country was placed in lockdown.

Therefore, at least from the end of February 2020 the UK should have started testing, contact tracing and isolating. Quarantine should have been enforced for anyone coming from abroad. Most importantly however, UK's borders should have been closed to limit further addition of the virus into communities. Irrespective of the R value in February 2020, if there had been effective action at this stage, it may have been possible to contain spread of the virus.

On 3rd March there were 51 cases of Covid-19. In the first week of March the number of cases increased from 26 to 206.

On 7th March the Prime Minister was at the Six Nations Rugby match between England and Wales at Twickenham where 80,000 fans had been in attendance. The PM was seen shaking hands with some players. This image took one back to the BSE crisis when John Selwyn Gummer was photographed with his daughter eating beef burgers.

On 8th March the Six Nations Rugby match between Scotland and France took place at Murrayfield Stadium in Edinburgh. Many French supporters were among the crowd of about 67,000 to see the match. On the same day France banned gatherings of more than 1000 people.

Cheltenham Gold Cup Festival opened on 10 March with about 60,000 people attending every afternoon. The Cheltenham Gold Cup itself was on 13th March 2020 when about 68,500 people attended. On 17th March 2020 lockdown was announced. Many would ask why this horse-racing festival was allowed to continue when the pandemic in the UK was silently gathering pace. The science was already there.

Again on 11th March the football match between the clubs, Liverpool and Athletico Madrid, went ahead with 52,000 supporters attending the match in Liverpool. This number included 3000 supporters from Madrid. Spain was suffering an increase in cases of Covid-19 at this time. On 14th March, Spanish Prime Minister, Pedro Sanchez, declared a state of emergency. This required people to stay at home in Spain to try and curb the spread of Covid-19. The number of cases of Covid-19 in Liverpool began to rise a week after the match. It was estimated that the football match at Liverpool and the Cheltenham horse races contributed to 41 and 37 extra deaths respectively in hospital.

Nor had Scotland done any better. A sportswear conference organised by Nike was held on 26th February in Edinburgh. This was attended by 70 delegates from around the world. At the same time the venue was also being used for an event by staff of Lloyds Bank. At least 25 persons were infected by the virus from one person who was carrying the infection. The public was kept in the dark about the matter. Lloyds Bank and those who transported the delegates to the conference were not informed of the carrier in their midst. The failure to disclose what had happened is at best a lack of candour and at worst a demonstration of scant regard for the health of the public.

The failure to contain spread of the virus is one important strand in any future review of why the UK fared so badly with Covid-19. It appears that the policy of government and supported by the scientific community was to allow herd immunity to develop. Herd immunity is not likely to develop in any infection unless large numbers get the infection and survive it. Or, if significant numbers of people are immunised against the infection. Immunisation against Covid-19 is not available. But it is surprising that the government maintained in June 2020 that herd immunity had never been its policy or goal in dealing with the pandemic. One has to ask why herd policy was mentioned in many public briefings at the outset in January and February if herd immunity was not an objective of the government. Alternatively one needs to know what the plan was at this stage. Sir Patrick Vallance said that 60% of the population would need to become infected for effective herd immunity. Thus the view was that 40 million people in the UK would have needed to become infected to attain meaningful herd immunity. The conclusion therefore seemed to be to allow as many to get infected while apparently protecting the vulnerable. If the aim was to increase herd immunity it is therefore a conclusion that a large number of deaths would have been acceptable among those who were not vulnerable. There would also need to have been extensive testing to ensure that the vulnerable were not in contact with anyone who could have been a carrier of the virus.

It is worrying to extrapolate from the 60% infection rate suggested in the preceding paragraph. A publication in the medical journal, Lancet of 12th March quoted a global mortality rate of 5.7% with a death rate as high as 20% in Wuhan where the infection started. Therefore the scientific advisers to the government were considering a death rate of 5.7% in the 40 million who would have needed to get the infection so as to provide meaningful herd immunity. Other figures quote a mortality of 1% of patients dying. At the time of this writing the death rate in UK was 14.1% while globally it was 6.3%. Using the lowest figure of 5.7%, it would have amounted to over two and a quarter million people dead in the UK! Even a rate of 1% would have meant 400,000 people dying of the infection. If one uses the death rate of 14% at the time of this writing, the UK would have had a colossal 5 million deaths. This is almost twenty times the combined deaths following the nuclear bombs dropped on Hiroshima and Nagasaki in August 1945.

On 12th March there were 596 cases and 10 people had died from the virus. On this day contact tracing was abandoned.

By this time other countries had acted differently. China, South Korea and Italy were in lockdown and schools were closed in Denmark, and in Ireland.

Sweden with a population of almost 10 million did not place the country in lockdown. It shared information with people, advised them about the nature of Covid-19 and relied on the public sense of duty to abide with advice. Social distancing was advised but schools, bars, restaurants etc were kept open. At the end of May, Sweden had 4468 deaths from Covid-19 compared to Norway's 237 (5. 4 million population), Finland 320 (population 5.5 million) and Denmark 580 (population 5.8 million). Yet 75,000 people have been made redundant and the economy of Sweden is likely to contract by 7% in 2020. This shows that even without lockdown the economy could not maintain its status quo. However, even in the absence of lockdown the infection rate in Sweden was less than the numbers in Spain, Italy and the UK. Could it have had a reduced death rate had lockdown been placed? It is possible that the death rate would have been less. But what we do not know in this pandemic is what other factors and actions were in play and were able to bear down to keep infections and death rates low.

Other countries like Singapore, Taiwan, Vietnam and South Korea acted swiftly to deal with the virus. Having been exposed to SARS they knew that time was of the essence. They introduced testing and tracing early. In the UK however the hope was that passive immunity would build up in the population and lead to effective herd immunity. This was based on the presumption that a large proportion of the population would get a 'mild' form of the disease and would develop protective antibodies. At that stage there was little information about the development of antibodies or how effective any antibodies were in protecting against infection. This was therefore a leap in the dark. Information on the effect of antibodies is still lacking; whether antibodies are produced in all who get the infection, how effective any antibodies are in protecting against further infection and how long they last in the human body are still unknown factors.

In comparison, New Zealand under Prime Minister Jacinda Arden adopted a 'precautionary approach'. Travellers to New Zealand from Italy were asked to self-isolate. The UK did not take any action although scientists warned that the virus was doubling every four to six days and there was the prospect that 80% of the population would have become infected. The government embarked on a contain, delay, research, mitigate strategy. There was a reluctance to move on to school closures, working from home etc due to what the government perceived was a balance between health and economics. This led to waiting. It would appear that in the early stages of the pandemic in the UK, the economic consequences of lockdown were given greater priority over people's health.

The effect on the elderly and those in care homes was not given the attention that it deserved. A priority was to protect the NHS. It was assumed that any surge in infections would have overwhelmed the NHS and may have severely curtailed its ability to care for patients. This happened in Italy and appears to have had a significant bearing on the decision to protect the NHS. That infection was occurring in the community and likely to lead to death and thereby put pressure on the NHS seems to have been either ignored or discounted. The NHS did cope admirably; this was undoubtedly due to the amazing commitment of staff, volunteers etc and to the cessation or postponement of other non-Covid related clinical activities.

The approach appears to have been to let everyone to contract the infection without any coordinated effort at suppressing spread of the virus. The fear of suppression was that the virus would emerge later, perhaps during the winter flu season with catastrophic effects on people and on the NHS. Therefore in the early stages, life appears to have been going on as normal. The silent killer in the midst was not seen as a potent threat as yet.

Many other countries were surprised at the approach the UK was taking. Beppe Severgnini, writing in the conservative Italian newspaper, Corriere della Sera, wrote that Britain had "lost the advantage that fate and Italy gave it – for example, the first two weeks of the outbreak in Italy when it was obvious the virus was spreading".

How well was the UK prepared, if an overwhelming pandemic were to affect it? How would the NHS contain spread of the virus? How would the public be protected?

When one reviews Europe as a whole and how the pandemic was being dealt with, it is not difficult to conclude that the situation in care homes was and continues to be the Achilles heel in containing spread of infection. Little attention appears to have been paid to what was happening in care homes. The elderly and the vulnerable became infected and contributed to about 40% of total deaths. Additionally care homes became the source from which spread of the virus occurred in the community. In trying to protect the NHS the elderly were placed at risk. Herein lies an important lesson for any government planning for a second wave or the next pandemic. The entire spectrum of health care needs to be surveyed and covered by precautionary measures. In default the problem moves from an area that is being protected to another area.

Let's look at Exercise Cygnus which took place in 2016. It was a massive exercise involving more than 950 people and included dummy COBRA meetings. This was as real as it could get and was done with the purpose of seeing if the UK could cope with a pandemic. This was a simulation of what would happen if the UK was affected by a flu pandemic. It was called a 'tactical exercise' done to test the resilience of the NHS, social care etc if the country had to deal with a pandemic of flu. The exercise involved many government departments that would feature in dealing with a pandemic. The scenario of the exercise was that even though the pandemic had not reached its peak there were not enough PPE, ventilators were in short supply and mortuaries were full of bodies. Following this exercise there was a long list of recommendations, which were not implemented. This had the effect of worsening the situation at a time that the government was preoccupied with Brexit and apparently took its eye off the pandemic. There was no contingency planning and the country was caught out unprepared.

Around the middle of February 2020, the government sent 1800 pairs of goggles, 194,000 wipes, 430,000 pairs of disposable gloves, 2500 face masks and 37,500 medical gowns to China, following an appeal from the country. Far from criticising the UK government for this, it is important to recognise that this was a necessary act of assistance at a time of need for China. To help another country combat the pandemic is a basic ethical act. Such an act not only helps the people of the receiving country but also, in the case of the pandemic, it is likely to reduce worldwide spread. Above all it is a humane act. China had since then supplied the UK with much more equipment to help us combat Covid-19. What is at issue however is the statement by Michael Gove, Minister for the Cabinet Office, that what was sent to China was 'not from our pandemic stock'. He challenged the impression that 'we've been running down stocks'. But we know that we did not have enough stock in reserve to deal with the pandemic, when it came to our shores. Equally important is that at this stage the UK government still did not perceive the coronavirus as a threat and appears to have continued with its belief of the infection being a mild condition that would induce antibodies and help raise the level of herd immunity.

The nation's supply of PPE was being depleted without the government reinforcing stocks. The government also did not contact the Healthcare Trades Association (HTA) for help in sourcing supplies to bolster its existing stocks. In another failure to obtain PPE, it is known that the HTA was asked to supply PPE only in April 2020. Often, PPE that was available was out of date and these were not replenished. The NHS Operating Framework for Managing the Response to Pandemic Influenza of 2017 talked about 'just in case contracts', should stockpiles fall below a critical level. It was often difficult if not impossible to activate these contracts. Most of these contracts were with Chinese suppliers. The latter were facing unprecedented demand from China itself and could not meet the needs of the UK. But then the NHS could have turned to UK suppliers. However, it did so only after 1st April; again an unnecessary delay.

In Exercise Cygnus, the social care system was expected to support the country in the event of a pandemic. What was worrying is that the impact of a pandemic on the country was not sufficiently appreciated in Whitehall. The report on Cygnus stated that; 'the UK's preparedness and response, in terms of its plans, policies and capability, is currently not sufficient to cope with the extreme demands of a severe pandemic…' The Health Secretary, Matt Hancock, claimed in April 2020 'everything that was appropriate to do was done'. We now know that the care home sector was not adequately prepared to deal with the pandemic. Residents in care homes are those at the highest risk for getting Covid-19 and the group that the government sought at the outset to protect the most. That this sector of the community was failed reflects an inadequacy in the scientific advice to government or in its application. Protection of the elderly and vulnerable in care homes would have needed not only social isolation but also testing of everyone who came in to the homes. This should have included those who worked in the care homes, suppliers to the homes etc. A rigidly enforced cordon sanitaire in homes would have protected this group of people. It would also have helped prevent care homes from being the sources of continued re-infection of the community with the virus.

Among the recommendations after Cygnus was an increase in the capacity of care homes and the numbers of staff who work in them. With prescience it warned about the challenges care homes would face when asked to accept patients form hospitals. Martin Green, the chief executive of Care England, said that 'It beggars belief, this is a report that made some really clear recommendations that haven't been implemented. If they had put in place a response to every one, we would have been in a much better place at the start of this pandemic.'

The NAO found that about 25,000 people were discharged from hospital into care homes between 17th March and 15th April 2020. It is not known how many of these people had Covid-19 at the time they were discharged into care homes. The need was to free up as many hospital beds as possible to enable hospitals to deal with any surge in cases of the infection. But the policy at the time was not to test all patients for Covid-19 before discharge into care homes. This was a period when there was an increase in the numbers of patients with positive Covid-19 and an increase in deaths from it. For e.g. on 11th April there were 9875 cases and 917 deaths. As the Chair of the Commons Health and Social Care Committee said' it seems extraordinary that no one appeared to consider the risks to care homes…'. The failure to test those being admitted to care homes would now be considered as a strategic error which contributed to the rise in cases and of deaths in care homes. The desire, quite rightly, to protect the NHS and retain capacity in it to deal with cases of Covid-19 led to a myopic view that prevented the Department of Health from seeing the looming crisis in care homes. This is all the more striking given the declared intention to protect the vulnerable. There could arguably be no greater vulnerable population than those in care homes.

The Care Quality Commission (CQC) oversees care of patients in care-homes in England, as it does of hospitals and other health care settings. It appears to have erred in not recognising the risks to residents of care homes from the policy of accepting patients discharged from hospitals without Covid-19 tests. It has apparently failed to act proactively and not alerted the Department of Health of the risks in discharging patients to homes.

But there is a need to place testing of patients prior to discharge of patients from hospitals into care homes in some perspective. It was often not possible in the early stages of the pandemic to get tests done even for patients in hospital. Testing would not always give a clear answer. Like with all tests, there is a false positive and a false negative rate. It is possible for a person to be negative on testing but still have the virus. Conversely it is possible to be positive on testing and yet not have the virus. These are the vagaries of doing any test. A patient who is falsely positive and therefore not discharged to a care home would be retained in hospital. The patient is now at risk not only of getting Covid-19 but also of contracting other hospital associated infections. And the patient who is falsely negative would give a false sense of security but be a risk to other residents in a care home. This brings another factor into the debate about testing – the need for sequential tests.

It would appear that at the heart of government there was a lack of oversight of the emerging threat from the pandemic. The National Security Council (NSC) oversees threats of any kind to the country. This does not only include military threats. Matters like cyber-threats, threats to national infrastructure, and pandemics fall within the umbrella of the NSC. As Ben Wallace, Defence Secretary, said a 'influenza pandemic could have the potential to cause hundreds of thousands of fatalities and cost the UK tens of billions of pounds". A sub-committee of the NSC was the Threats, Hazards, Resilience and Contingency Committee (THRCC) that included Health Secretary Matt Hancock, current Minister for the Cabinet Office Michael Gove and Gavin Williamson who was Secretary of State for Defence. THRCC was chaired by the then Deputy Prime Minster David Liddington. Theresa May was Prime Minister at the time.

The THRCC was suspended by Theresa May in November 2018 due to pressures of dealing with Brexit. This was done on the advice of the then Cabinet Secretary, Sir Mark Sedwill. As a former Cabinet minister said "We had to spend more time on the EU exit strategy and less on everything else; it was felt that if we were going to get our ducks in a row to prepare for the risk of a no-deal scenario we had to slow down on things including THRCC".

THRCC was abolished by Boris Johnson in 2019 when he assumed office as Prime Minister. This may turn out to have been another significant strategic error in the preparation for the pandemic that eventually hit the UK. The threat of Covid-19 and its alarming spread in Italy were either not realised early or was considered minimal. THRCC could have been resurrected in time if the country had taken a more balanced view of the threats posed by the virus and followed the events that were unfolding in Italy. Time and again one is left asking what the scientific advice at the time was.

There was also a Resilience Capabilities Programme (RCP) which was managed by the Civil Contingencies Secretariat (CCS). In any subsequent inquiry into the pandemic in the UK, it would be as interesting as informative to understand the role of all the organisations which had responsibility for foreseeing and therefore acting to ameliorate the effects of the pandemic in the UK.

Here was an orchestra sans an effective conductor!

One could go further backwards in time to 2007 when another exercise, Winter Willow, took place. This massive exercise involved 5000 people from government, industry, voluntary sector etc to check how well the country was prepared to deal with a flu pandemic. The exercise was held in two stages, the first in January and the second in February 2007. It was recognised in this exercise that the Department of Health would work with the NHS to identify a range of essential health supplies and to look at the options to ensure continuity of availability of these items. This would include the availability of medicines and appliances that patients need as part of their on-going health care. Obtaining supplies of antibiotics and anti-viral medicines would be a priority.

Finally one has the UK's Pandemic Preparedness Plan of 2011 (PPP) which was based on a 'reasonable worst case' scenario. As we have been continuously informed and reminded during the Covid-19 crisis, government was planning for a worst case scenario while hoping for the best. This Plan noted that, regardless of where or when an influenza epidemic or pandemic started, it is likely to reach the UK very quickly. Also the appearance of a large number of cases over a short period of time would have a great impact on the public and on the ability of the NHS to manage the clinical situation. The same number of cases appearing over a longer period in time would be easier to manage. So it is easy to appreciate why the government was preparing for the peak of the illness, knowing that the UK was some weeks behind Italy in this respect. In Italy the peak of the infection caused a spike in deaths and was, to say the least, a huge burden on local health services. It is also easy to see why the Nightingale Hospitals were commissioned. This was good planning because, at the stage they were being constructed, it was not known how many cases there would be at the peak of the pandemic. Those who criticise the use of resources in the Nightingale Hospitals may have missed the crucial factor in their commissioning; the plan was to avoid the situation where demand for health care services outstripped the ability of the NHS to provide services that are needed for Covid-19 patients and generally. What would have happened if there was a great surge in cases of Covid-19 which overwhelmed the NHS and especially its availability of intensive care and ventilation to patients who needed them? One could imagine a scenario where some patients would have to have ventilation denied them - a sort of 'medical, ethical and moral lottery'. That the Nightingale Hospitals were not used to full capacity and that NHS intensive care facilities were able to manage the demand is a tribute to the services in the NHS and to the prior planning for any excess capacity that may have been required. This part of the PPP also explains why the NHS slogans of the time spoke of 'Save the NHS'. If the NHS was overwhelmed by Covid-19 patients and there was reduction in staff due to the same illness or contact related isolation, there was the possibility that many more than Covid-19 patents would have suffered.

The tragedy with the PPP was that it was good for the purpose, but not implemented. Professor Martin Hibberd of the London School of Hygiene and Tropical Medicine (LSHTM) compared the performance of the UK with that of Singapore, which had used the UK's PPP. Singapore was successful in containing the virus because they had implemented the plan. The UK did not and paid the price with rising infection and increasing numbers who died.

It is accepted that an influenza pandemic is unpredictable - in the nature of the infection, the rate of its spread, the types of people affected, who would die from it and the response of patients to any treatment that is available. It is also unpredictable in terms of the demands it makes on a country's health and social care systems. The PPP noted that during the pandemic any response to it will be influenced by available information and evidence that may emerge at the time. Now, this is interesting in the current situation. As regards timing, the UK was behind the overwhelming epidemic that affected Italy. We also know how other countries were managing the pandemic, especially how South Korea and New Zealand dealt with the risk of the virus in their countries. The UK did not consider it necessary to test for the virus. Nor did it see the need for sustained contact tracing. Contact tracing was terminated about mid-March. At the outset the Director General of WHO, Tedros Adhanom Ghebreyusus, said 'Test, Test, Test'. The reasoning behind this was to identify those who had infection and to focus the initial contact tracing from here. Isolation of these persons at an early stage is likely to have limited the spread of infection. Experts from the Universities of Cambridge and Manchester produced a report on 12th February advising a ten-fold increase in the test and trace capacity of Public Health England. The government's Chief Scientific Advisor, Sri Patrick Vallance and its Chief Medical Officer, Chris Whitty, stated on 27th February that the top priority should be to 'detect and monitor any outbreak as effectively as possible'.

Although testing was crucial it appears that both Public Health England and the Care Quality Commission obstructed any progress in this respect. Staff needed to perform tests were required to have been appropriately trained and accredited. All this, to be able to insert a swab into another person's nose or throat. The country was facing a crisis and the organisations whose responsibility it was to protect the public failed to rise up to the challenge. As a result, residents of care homes, who were those at greatest risk, were denied early testing. The CQC claimed that the tests needed to be done correctly by appropriately trained personnel and that residents needed to provide full consent. By the latter it is presumed that all residents had to provide fully informed consent. Of course some test results would come back negative due to faulty procedure or the natural false negative and false positive rates of the test. This is common with any test. But the delay in testing for the reasons given above was to delay diagnosis and to permit spread of Covid-19 in care homes. This is what eventually happened.

The government was slow in rolling out testing and some like public health specialist, Professor Helen Ward of Imperial College, London said in April that 'politicians refused to listen to advice' on testing. Testing and tracing was stopped because PHE did not have the capacity to manage the program. As at 18th February PHE could only test five Covid-19 cases a week! SAGE agreed that suspending test and trace was 'sensible' while the CMO, Prof. Chris Whitty said that ceasing routine testing on 5th March was because there was only a 'slim to zero' chance that a global pandemic would be averted. This was the time the deputy CMO, Dr.Jenny Harries said that 'there comes a point in a pandemic where that is not an appropriate intervention'. Professor Yvonne Doyle, PHE's medical director, told MPs the decision was to focus testing on the NHS and to stop community testing and tracing. This underlines the fact that the NHS was the priority and protecting it was vital to the health of the nation. While this is undoubtedly an appropriate view, it ignored the looming crisis in the community and in care homes. These statements did not take account of public concern and the need to reassure by having a satisfactory testing program in place. 'Test, Test, Test' were the words of the DG, Dr.Tedros while the WHO claimed that countries were not doing enough testing. The government's CSA, Sir Patrick Vallance, was of the view that failure to test was one of the major errors in UK's handling of the pandemic. The Government's consistent position at the time was that they were following scientific advice.

A member of SAGE, Jeremy Farrar said that ceasing testing was a mistake. Testing should have been commenced early and done across all sectors- hospital, community and care homes. Additionally he stressed that lockdown restrictions only be lifted when the test and trace program was in place.

Failure to have an effective test and trace program was the reason UK had a high death rate from Covid-19.

Professor Ward was even harder in her comments, continuing 'they decided they knew better; there will be reckoning and it will not be forgiving'.

The advice to test and trace was jettisoned in the middle of March

2020. It is not known why Public Health England decided not to follow, what turned out to be the successful test and trace system used by South Korea.

It is not always possible to accept assurances made by government that it was following scientific advice. Test and trace was jettisoned despite Sir Patrick Vallance and Prof Chris Whitty stating at the SAGE meeting of 27th February that the main priority was to 'detect and monitor any outbreak as effectively as possible'. This could never be achieved in the absence of testing. Therefore it appears that a significant aspect of scientific advice was ignored. Additionally this was an important foundation in the ability to control the pandemic.

Towards the end of April with a target set for 100,000 tests a day, the UK had the lowest rate of testing in Europe. The UK's test rate was 5.54 per 100 people compared with the highest in Iceland of 124. The deputy Chief Medical Officer, Jenny Harries implied that there was no clear link between more testing and a lower death rate.

Testing and tracing with isolation when needed, in care homes would have limited infection especially with the need to accept patients who were discharged from hospitals. The Department of Health advised that care homes take in patients discharged from hospital to free hospital bed capacity. Some of these were likely to be Covid-19 patients while others would not have had any tests for the virus. Naturally, the care home sector was up in arms about this decision because of the risk of spreading the virus even further in homes. This policy coupled with the dearth of PPE put untold pressure on care homes. At one point in the middle of April a quarter of the residents in care homes in Sheffield were infected and thirty care staff were positive on testing for Covid-19. Residents were confined to their rooms with no family or visitors allowed. This was at a time when the Chancellor of the Exchequer said that residents of care homes and those who worked in them would not be forgotten. But the figures tell a different story. For example, HC-One is the UK's biggest care home provider which has several care homes in and around London and others located around the four nations of the UK. In April, HC-One had about 1500 cases of the infection spread across its 233 care homes. The number who had died from Covid-19 was 311. MHA Care Homes, another big provider had Covid-19 in half of its 131 care homes.

The UK had already seen and heard about the crisis facing other European countries like Italy and Spain. The UK was several weeks behind these countries and so had time to prepare, not only the hospital sector but also the vulnerable residents and their carers in care homes. It was known that up to 50% of deaths from Covid-19 were in care homes.

Department of Health guidelines indicated that some patient sent to care homes may have Covid-19, even if they did not have symptoms. Transferring patients into care homes without testing was labelled 'crimes against the elderly'. Managers of several care homes refused to comply with guidance as they could see that residents would have been placed at risk. What was ridiculous was that at the same time that residents were being put at risk by admission of untested patients, relatives of residents already in homes were prevented from visiting their loved ones even with PPE.

Here lies a good example of failure of the system to contain the virus and reduce the death toll. Testing should have been introduced early into care homes. This is where the most vulnerable section of the population lives in close proximity to each other. This was shielding in the community but totally different to shielding at home. Here the vulnerable were not shielded from those who may have Covid-19 or from the risk of cross infection due to the lack of testing, lack of PPE etc. This was no shielding at all! These were the real lambs to the slaughter. Deaths in care homes contributed to a quarter of Covid-19 related deaths in Scotland.

The Care Quality Commission (CQC) which oversees adult health and social care had been informed about the discharge policy of hospitals. Patients were being discharged into care homes without testing, placing residents and staff of the homes at risk. The CQC's head for adult social care said it was looking at whether hospital had breached their duty of care and whether the CQC was in a position to take action against the hospitals. This is a ridiculous position to take. What action could the CQC take without jeopardising the care being provided by hospitals and putting even more lives at risk? While the CQC could enforce certain steps that hospitals would have been compelled to take, these were not likely in the middle of a crisis. CQC had not anticipated the risks and had not been proactive. It too could be held responsible for sleep-walking into the crisis. It would have been aware of the Pandemic Preparedness Plan and should have held the Health Service to account regarding stockpiles, discharges etc. While the CQC claims that it helped care homes in securing PPE etc, the fact remains that it did not act at the outset to protect them. The CQC appears to have supported the policy of the Department of Health to discharge people, from hospitals to care homes. It should have intervened early to ensure that only those who tested negative to the coronavirus were allowed in to care homes. This would have helped stem infection of residents and carers and thereby reduced the spread of infection. Many residents died alone with no contact from family and loved ones. This must be the saddest saga of the pandemic in the UK.

The Good Law Project (GLP) is a not-for-profit membership organisation that serves the interest of the public. It uses the existing law to defend what it perceives to be right and hold to account those who appear to be in breach of the law. GLP heard of a Hospital Trust that had issued guidance to its doctors to avoid using Covid-19 as a cause of death in Medical Certificates of Cause of Death (MCCD). A MCCD has the main causes listed in 1a of the form with subsidiary or contributory causes listed thereafter in lines 1b and 1c. The Trust had advised doctors who were filling in MCCD's to use 'Pneumonia' or 'Community Acquired Pneumonia' as the primary cause of death in 1a of the form. The Trust advised doctors that there is no requirement to state Covid-19 on a MCCD. But it also advised that a doctor may add Covid-19 in 1b of the MCCD, if the doctor so wished. On the face of it, this advice appears to seek to reduce the numbers of reported deaths in the Trust from Covid-19. This would have the effect of diminishing the total numbers who died of Covid-19 in the hospital but it would also have reduced the total number of deaths reported regionally and nationally. GLP sought legal advice and wrote to the Trust, who withdrew the guidance. It also undertook a review of MCCD's that had been issued since the guidance was in use.

Initially the UK used quarantine for about 300 persons. This included about 80 persons who were repatriated form Wuhan and another 30 from the cruise ship, the Diamond Princess which was docked in Yokohama, Japan. But this policy was abandoned soon afterwards. About 1.8 million people arrived in the UK between 1st January and 25th March 2020. These people came from all around the world. Of this total of passengers, about 275 who came from China and Japan were taken into quarantine. Of the rest of the passengers who arrived it is not known how many had the infection and how many of them had chosen to self isolate if they had symptoms. Had there been screening, at the ports of entry, for at least a raised temperature, it is possible that some spread would have been avoided. It is accepted that no single preventive action alone and of itself would have limited the spread of Covid-19 in UK. Containing spread depends on many small gains.

South Korea and Singapore used testing and contact tracing effectively. South Korea's foreign minister, Kang Kyung-wha, said that her country developed testing early on and used it widely. This no doubt helped to limits the number of cases in her country.

Hong Kong also acted early and informed doctors to be alert to patients presenting with chest symptoms especially those who had been to China. Also on 30th January it shut down the rail link between Hong Kong and Wuhan. The habit of wearing masks had become commonplace after the SARS epidemic of 2002. The combination of the use of face marks, testing and tracing, border restriction and some social distancing have been effective in Hong Kong. It had just over a 1000 cases of Covid-19 and only 4 deaths in a population of 7.3 million people. These are remarkable figures given the proximity of Hong Kong to mainland China and the links between the two countries. Hong Kong also has a high level of interconnectivity, being an important transport hub.

Many countries shut their borders to prevent the spread of Covid-19. New Zealand, for example, closed its borders on 19th March. The PPP recognised that because of the UK's 'high level of international connectivity', a pandemic is likely to affect the UK early. This did not happen as we were behind Italy by a few weeks. This time lag provided an opportunity to put in practice any plan to combat the infection. Modelling suggested that a 90% restriction on all air travel to the UK would delay the pandemic by one or two weeks. The same models suggest that a 99.9% of reduction of travel would have delayed the peak of the pandemic by two months. Why border restrictions were not put in place is a source of much debate, especially knowing that other countries have done so effectively.

Vietnam had suffered from previous epidemics and knew that action was needed as soon as it was aware of Covid-19. After recognising eight cases of the virus infection it instituted lockdown, compared to the UK which did so after several thousand cases had been reported. Vietnam has a population of 30 million, about half that of the UK. Vietnam had 271 cases and no deaths. Although there are concerns about the accuracy of the figures, most agree that the disease is low in Vietnam. It was able to do this by being aggressive in its use of lockdown - almost a curfew. This is easy to achieve in a communist state like Vietnam or in a dictatorship, but not acceptable in a liberal democracy. However, Vietnam's effectiveness in containing the pandemic is impressive. So effective was its action that Vietnam was considering easing lockdown in the end of April 2020.

It is interesting to compare the performance of eastern and western Europe in combating the infection. One cannot entirely disagree with the view expressed by Slawomir Debski, director of the Polish Institute of International Affairs who wrote "in the West people believed that high-tech societies with very good health care could deal with anything, and that created an illusion that they would have the time and the tools to fight a sudden pandemic'.

The initial response of the government was on containment. However containment can only go so far. Containment in 2009 of the H1N1 influenza epidemic failed. There was no chance that this policy would work with a global pandemic. It appears that time was wasted.

The PPP described how, during the swine flu pandemic of 2009, the virus had spread widely before international health authorities were alert to its presence and its ability to spread. PPP uses this as an argument against closing borders. But the UK had information from what was happening in China and in Italy to help it to act early to contain the virus. The view expressed in the PPP that 'economic, political and social consequences of border control would be very substantial' appears untenable. The reduction in movement of people was crucial to containing the virus. Movements of goods, pharmaceuticals, healthcare supplies, food etc would not be disrupted so long as these activities continued in accordance with social distancing and other general health advice. As it happened, international air travel largely came to a standstill. In the UK British Airways, Virgin, Easyjet and Ryanair ceased flights.

Even as late as the beginning of May 2020 it was estimated that up to 15,000 people were arriving in the UK from Italy, China and Iran. There were no checks at the airport, no body temperature check and no quarantine. The passengers were simply handed information leaflets. We do not know how many people with infection came into the country during lockdown. We do not know the extent of addition to the pool of infected people in the UK. With the R number under 1, it remained important to test, screen and isolate to keep R as low as possible.

Belatedly there was an announcement around 27th April that arrivals to the UK would be quarantined. Singapore, for e.g., enforced travel restrictions from the outset while the UK largely remained lax in this respect. Except for some examples of quarantine, people were subsequently allowed to travel in to the country without any checks being made. This undoubtedly added to the pool of infection in the country by helping the virus to spread.

Even China enforced a travel ban with thermal imaging of body temperature of arrivals. The UK was trying to close the door tool late in the infection. Yet it is never late to stop or at least reduce the impact of a second wave of the virus, if it occurs. What is difficult to understand is whether scientific advice in the UK differed from that available in other countries like Australia, New Zealand and Germany. These countries all ended with much lower numbers of the infection and much less deaths in their populations. It would be useful in any subsequent inquiry into the pandemic in the UK to understand the scientific evidence that was provided to government. It would, also help to appreciate how much of the evidence stood up to scrutiny compared to similar evidence used in other countries. In the final analysis, like in war, decisions have to be made politically, not by generals or scientists. The dilution or modification, if any, of evidence to meet economic and political imperatives would shed interesting light on how government weighed up priorities in its final decisions.

Lockdown was a necessity, despite its adverse economic impact, among others. What is in question is the timing of it.

Unfortunately the delay in acting was seen again when lockdown was re-imposed in Leicester in June 2020. At the end of June the infection rate in Leicester was 140 cases per 100,000 of the population compared to Bradford which was 69 cases per 100,000 of population at the same time. A week later Leicester's rate had gone up to 141 while that in Bradford had fallen to 46. The reasons for this increase in infection was due to people in Leicester not complying with lockdown advice and to the overcrowded working conditions in some of the businesses in the Leicester. There were businesses that apparently continued to work throughout the period of the original lockdown. The emerging problems in Leicester were known to the government on 8th June and a related public health meeting was held on 15th June. A team was sent from Public Health England to Leicester only on 26th June and the order to lockdown was finally signed by the Prime Minister on 29th June. Yet again procrastination and bureaucracy led to delay, with the virus spreading in the intervening period between identifying the issues and the order to lockdown finally being signed.

There was no drive to develop a test for Covid-19 or to test widely. We learn that the government did not seek the help of UK diagnostic test manufacturers until 1st April 2020.

The Pandemic Preparedness Plan described the importance of the public in managing a pandemic. Individual responsibility, care for self and supporting neighbours, community etc. In lockdown we have seen how the vast majority of people have complied with restrictions in their lives and made the most of staying at home.

While New Zealand's remote location in the world and small population helped it to contain the virus, these factors alone do not explain its success. Irrespective of population size and location New Zealand is as interconnected as most other countries. New Zealand succeeded because it robustly contained transmission by testing, tracing and isolating contacts. Borders were sealed early and all those who arrived in New Zealand went into quarantine.

In 2007 Nassim Nicholas Taleb published 'The Black Swan'. In this book he talks of the Black Swan as a random event. It is an event that does not fit into the usual expectations or calculations of reasonable and rational human beings. We like our graphs and plots of the past to help us predict the future. These also help in, for e.g., mathematical modelling. There is nothing wrong with these. It is just as well to also remember what is, for e.g., in the small print. Like when we seek to invest money – it says 'past performance is no guarantee of future results'. What this means is that what happened before is not guaranteed to happen again or if such occurs, that it would follow a similar trajectory. Yet all these events, whatever forms they may take when they recur, have a similar theme but vary in details. These are the opposite of the random event which is the Black

Swan. The Black Swan describes the uselessness of previous knowledge when a random event occurs. There are no previous human experiences to fall back on when confronted with a truly random event. Such an event is totally unexpected; management of the event has to start from scratch and find one's way as one progresses. In some respects the total lockdown of the UK and especially in a bustling, vibrant city like London is a Black Swan. One could never have expected London to fall silent. Even during the blitz of World War 2, most people went about their normal lives.

However, Covid-19 was not a Black Swan. Far from it! The scientific information published in reputable journals has shown that there are bats which are a rich reservoir of coronaviruses. These viruses are changing (mutating) all the time. And the possibility of transmission to human beings is acknowledged. It happened with SARS. Why could not it happen again – indeed why should it not happen again, as it has done with Covid-19. And, here is the most worrying aspect of it all. There are many more coronaviruses awaiting the right conditions to infect and spread among human beings.

That the government has NERVTAG (New and Emerging Respiratory Virus Threats Advisory Group (NERVTAG) and a Pandemic Preparation Plan are tacit acknowledgement that the risk of a pandemic was taken seriously. Why was the advice from these plans and groups not heeded?

In the initial period the perceived wisdom was that herd immunity would help to contain the virus. This was also the view held in Sweden. On the 23rd of March, however, the government in the UK brought in lockdown. Sweden on the other had carried on without lockdown. People in Sweden acted sensibly, maintaining a social distance and working as far as possible from home. At the time of writing Sweden, with a population of nearly 10 million people, had 30,143 cases and 3679 deaths from Covid-19. So compared to Sweden, the numbers of cases and deaths per million of the population is higher in the UK with lockdown. The density of a city like London, the numbers of arrivals from abroad, the issues in care homes etc are likely to have contributed to the higher rate in the UK. Perhaps these figures make a case for having had more drastic action earlier than we did. Even Sweden acknowledged that it had erred by not having restrictions and that it's experiment with 'freedom' had failed.

The scientific community knew that SARS had come from bats. They also knew that it was a matter of time before a significant epidemic or pandemic happened, as we are now seeing with Covid-19. And they knew that human-to-human transmission was always likely to happen. With these facts known as recently as 2018 it is astonishing that in the UK, scientists did not take the risks more seriously in early January 2020. Or did they, but advise was diluted or even ignored in some instances? By the same token it was undiplomatic for the Work and Pensions Secretary Therese Coffey to have said that minsters received 'wrong' scientific advice about care homes. She went on 'I'm not surprised if people then think we made a wrong decision.' The public needed clearer information about how the situation, as it evolved, was being managed. The, physicist Professor Brian Cox said it was not enough for minsters to say that they were "following the science'. The public needs to know what the scientific advice was at the time and how it was used to fashion policy. People accept that this is a rapidly evolving situation and that there were no correct answers. Policy needed to be modified in response to the changing scenario. The public can judge for themselves and would credit politicians if there was no ideal solution so long as they knew the underlying scientific information and appreciated that this was also qualified and limited.

According to Professor Devi Sridhar the UK squandered the head start it had to deal effectively with Covid-19. Gabriel Scally from the University of Bristol, Bobbie Jacobson from John Hopkins University and Kamran Abbasi, Executive Editor of the British Medical Journal wrote 'By the time the UK formally announced a lockdown with a huge package of economic support measures, almost two months of potential preparation and prevention time were squandered.'

We have managed epidemics well in the past. We have to learn from the current crisis and resolve to do better when we are next in a similar situation. In the words of the CQC, UK's Public Health Service and pandemic management 'Requires Improvement'.

o0:0o

BARBED WIRE DISEASE

What is this thing called 'lockdown'?
Quarantine and lockdown have been used to contain and manage epidemics and pandemics ever since the Justinian Plague which affected the Byzantine Empire, its capital of Constantinople and the Sasanian Empire. The Sasanian Empire was the last pre-Islam Iranian empire. It is called the Justinian plague after emperor Justinian (482AD- 565AD) who was ruler of Byzantium. Justinian himself got the plague, caused by the germ *Yersina pestis* which probably came from China and other parts of the Far East. Justinian survived the plague unlike the Athenian general Pericles (495BC - 429BC) who succumbed to it.

Lockdown is not a prison, but it is a prison of sorts. One cannot go out of the house, but one can do so for some specific reasons. One is told that it is being done for one's good and the good of others; like the phrase 'correctional facility' one encounters in the USA. In lockdown the 'correction' sought is control and eventual elimination of the infection.

But, and this is the important difference with a 'correctional facility', one has not been accused of and deemed guilty of any wrong doing. Lockdown is instituted to prevent one getting an illness that invisibly exists in one's midst. It cannot be seen but others may have it and pass it to you. You may contract the virus, get ill and be admitted to hospital. In hospital one may need complex labour-intensive treatments including oxygen and ventilation. You may pass the infection on to others and so perpetuate the infection. All of these events may put any healthcare system under considerable strain. You are asked to stay at home and save life and the NHS.

So for now, home is one's prison. That is what lockdown has done – converted my home, my castle into my prison.

For the vast majority of us prison is a place one hears about in the news or occasionally sees while driving past one. One may notice the high walls, barbed wire on the perimeter and the metal entrance doors with guards. It is soon forgotten as our attention moves to the next topic. Few indeed would stop and reflect on what it is like to be in a prison. What goes on inside a prison? More importantly what goes on in the mind of a prisoner?

Prison is a place most of us would choose not to go into; certainly not to be an inmate of. Some have written about their experience of being prisoners. Jonathan Aitken, a previous Member of Parliament (MP) and a cabinet minister in the UK government wrote about some aspects of his life in prison. He was convicted of perjury in 1999 and sentenced to prison for 18 months. He served seven months of his sentence. There is no doubt that prison had a profound impact on him. It is reported that while in prison he joined a prayer group which included murderers. He studied theology after being released from prison and was ordained as deacon. He continued thereafter to work in prison. He wrote about the problems of drugs in prison and that a significant proportion of prisoners tend to re-offend on release.

In his writing, Jonathan Aitken was drawing attention to the despair that surrounds most prisoners.

In legally enforced house arrest a person is confined to their homes and not permitted to go out or they could only go out under specific conditions, like for medical care. In criminal cases, house arrest could be enforced by electronic tagging of the individual. The electronic tag would allow authorities to monitor the individual and ensure that they stay confined to their homes. Some repressive regimes could use house arrest as a means of suppressing dissent. House arrest could come with other limitations for e.g. the person may be barred from using the internet and prevented from associating with other persons. Even telephone conversations may be monitored. All of these acts amount to severe censorship of the individual; it is imprisonment outside the confines of a traditional prison. Some national leaders who had spent time under house arrest were General

Augusto Pinochet of Chile, Aung San Suu Kyi of Myanmar and Imran Khan the current Prime Minister of Pakistan. Even Galileo Galilei was placed under house arrest for supporting Copernicus's theory that the earth rotated around the sun. Galileo died while under house arrest; he was eventually proven right and the Catholic Church wrong! In all cases of house arrest there was an immediate purpose that appeared to have been served by the detention of the individual at home.

In the UK, house arrest is sometimes used as a stepping-stone towards the early release of some offenders and to help them re-integrate into society. Early release also helps to reduce overcrowding in prisons and to contain costs of running the prison system.

When lockdown was introduced, the Daily Telegraph wrote 'End of Freedom", while the Financial Times claimed that the Prime Minister was forced to close Britain.

The Star newspaper of 24th March screamed- 'Your Country Needs You… to Naff Off Home' with a picture of Lord Kitchener of Khartoum and his famous pointing index finger. The message was clear – go home and stay at home!

While some would maintain that lockdown and legal house arrest are much the same; this is not so. A person who is subject to house arrest is there as punishment for a wrong that was done. He had been judged to need punishment in the form of being under house arrest. Political prisoners are in a similar category; they have offended by their actions or views, the prevailing law of the time, whether the latter was justified or not. Also whether their acts were of sufficient severity to need house arrest is often debatable. Lockdown as we know it in UK today is not being done as a form of punishment. On the contrary it is being done for your good and for the greater good of society in curbing the spread of infection with the coronavirus. Some would try to convince us that a wrongdoer is under house arrest also for the greater good of society. Yes – but house arrest is punitive for wrongs done. Far from being punitive, lockdown brings into sharp contrast how interconnected and interdependent we are in a way that few of us had hitherto encountered or even imagined.

Stay at home was the message of the time because as the Prime Minister said 'this is a national emergency'. This is the first time since World War

2 when people were incarcerated in their homes for their own good. Then it was a military enemy, now it is a microbial one, a virus.

Of course lockdown needs to be accepted by the population. Therefore it is not surprising that it fell on the Police to ensure that lockdown was respected and that breach of lockdown regulations did not occur. So it was that we saw on TV, police patrolling parks, beaches and other communal areas, encouraging the public to return home and to stay there.

There were reports of police using roadblocks, checkpoints and drones to enforce the lockdown. House parties, barbecues etc were broken up. In one instance a pub was forced shut by police. They responded to a tip-off that people were drinking in the Pitsmoor Hotel in Sheffield. When police turned up at the pub in the hotel, they found people even hiding in cupboards to avoid being caught!

Although none of us would voluntarily agree to become a prisoner, most do not realize that we not infrequently become 'prisoners' ourselves without realizing what is happening. It is sometimes said that two not uncommon prisoners outside a traditional prison are those who are prisoners of their own thoughts and those who are prisoners within the walls of their homes. To be a prisoner of one's thoughts is to be in what seems to be an inescapable prison. One cannot run away from thoughts – they follow us where we go. Prisoners of their own thoughts arise from any one or more of the vicissitudes of life – financial, matrimonial or relationship, occupation or loss of it, family issues, bereavement etc. Each of these life events imposes a mental burden on the person. It or they occupy most of his time and are seen by the person, initially at least, as insuperable. Escape from it seems impossible for the person and they adversely affect work, interactions with others, sleep, appetite etc. They not infrequently lead to anxiety and depression of varying degrees. Resolving the worries brings relief and a welcome exit from this particular mental prison. But resolution is not always possible. Time heals; but how long is time? Seeing a counselor helps one to navigate a way through this apparently impenetrable maze. Often instead of resolution there is a useful degree of accommodation with and working around the problem. This arrangement brings a degree of peace.

Being a prisoner in one's home is a different situation. Common reasons why some people cannot leave their homes is physical disability or advanced aged and frailty. Loneliness at home is the desperate plight of many senior citizens in the UK. Confined to homes with little or no means of transport, they yearn for human contact and for contact with the outside world. Late autumn and winter are the most difficult times of the year for those at home; shorter periods of daylight and long dark evenings make the home a worse prison than it usually is to those who are confined to home. Lockdown has given the rest of society an insight to how the elderly and house-bound people probably lead their lives and cope with daily isolation. It has made us more aware of the quality of their lives. It is equally hoped that our experience of lockdown would move many of us to extend a helping hand to the lonely people in our society.

If one has suffered from, or currently suffers from or knows someone with agoraphobia one may understand what the fear of leaving home means. Agoraphobia is a complex mental condition which refers not only to a fear of open spaces. It may include a fear of leaving home. Home then becomes a prison for the person.

Much as we love our homes and feel secure in them, we need to go out of it to recognize its value to us. How often has one gone on holiday and yearned to be back home!

But when one is compelled to stay at home and not go out of it, home soon becomes a prison. It ceases to be the place where we long to return to, because we have not been away from it. It has now changed to a prison. When one is deprived of the freedom to come home and / or to leave it as and when one wished, home assumes a different character; it is no more one's home. And like any prison it causes you to behave differently towards it than you would otherwise have done. This 'home prison' causes anger, anxiety, frustration and a desire to return to normal days of before.

Covid -19 lockdown has made our homes 'prisons' and made us 'prisoners' in our own homes. This is the first time since the World War II that the public has had to endure some degree of 'incarceration' or 'curfew' designed to keep us at home against our will and for our own good.

One may also compare lockdown with quarantine. Many would ask what the difference between the two is. And lockdown lasts longer than quarantine. Quarantine is as old as human history. In the Old Testament, Leviticus states that people with leprosy needed to be outside the limits of the city. The plagues that afflicted Europe in the 14th century led to the deaths of about a third of the European population or 25 million people. It is possible that the word quarantine arose around this time. In 1374 Viscount Bernabo in Italy declared that persons with plague be taken out of the city and left in the fields to either die or recover. In Ragusa, which is Dubrovnik in Croatia today, a law was passed in 1377 preventing people from entering it from a plague infected area for a period of 30 days. During this period the people would remain in isolation, a *trentino* isolation period. The period of isolation was extended in later years to 40 days, a *quarantino* isolation period. The Italian word 'quaranta' means forty. It is uncertain why the forty day period was chosen. It may have been related to a Greek concept of a forty–day incubation period or 'critical days' before an infection caused symptoms. Or it may have been an arbitrary choice to reflect biblical events. All of this is interesting because they preceded the germ theory of disease by five hundred years. The germ theory of disease only arose in the nineteenth century with the work of Louis Pasteur (1822–95) and Ignaz Semmelweis (1818–65). The germ theory recognised for the first time germs as a cause of disease. Simmelweis wrote a book *'The Etiology, Concept, and Prophylaxis of Childbed Fever'* about the deaths of women from infection called puerperal infection or now called puerperal sepsis which was caused by germs. Puerperal sepsis was infection which occurs in mothers after giving birth, in the period called the puerperium. Another book by Irvine Loudon 'The Tragedy of Childbed Fever' describes details of maternal infection and death and the work of Simmelweis. Childbed fever was the commonest cause of death of women associated with childbirth in Britain before the Second World War. Poor hand washing was recognised as an important factor in the death of women, caused by the transmission of germs. Here we are in 2020 still extolling the virtues of hand-washing with soap and water to reduce the onward transmission of Covid-19.

To try to understand how people cope with and what happens to them during lockdown, it is probably interesting and useful to consider how prisoners of war (PoW's) coped in World War 1. When the Armistice was agreed in 1918 there were about 7 million prisoners of war held by Britain and Germany. At the end of World War II there were about 175,000 British prisoners held by the Germans and Italians. The prisoners had been in camps for varying periods of time, some for up to five years. One of the things that concerned the POW's was how long they would be in captivity.

In this respect, at least, it is not different to our current predicament; we do not know how long lockdown would continue for. The prison camps were cramped, with sparse rations and none of the home comforts that most of us have in lockdown. Not for them were smartphones, TV, Zoom and the like!

PoW's never expected to be captured. They would be back from the front, so they thought when they set out. We too never expected lockdown. Even the week before we moved into lockdown life went on as normal. The virus was elsewhere! When lockdown came, it brought with it the realisation that anyone of us could be affected and that some would die. The Prime Minister reminded us that we could lose loved ones before the pandemic was over. Suddenly it was real, unsettling and frightening. And it was severely disruptive of home, employment and careers, education of children, finances etc. Not even the financial crisis of 2008 affected all aspects of our lives suddenly and simultaneously and with such a great impact as lockdown 2020 does.

One important difference between PoW's and us in 2020 is that we have continuous updates from the government. There are also regular analyses of information in the newspapers and on television. This facility was not available to POW's who depended on little packets of information shared by other prisoners. The veracity of the information was questionable and it is likely that most of it consisted of rumour and speculation. PoW's were in an era of darkness that we cannot imagine. We are continuously submerged in a plethora of information that we have at our finger-tips and which we receive in real time. This is not to say that such information is always useful. It can be confusing and not infrequently one could not see the wood for the trees. Opinions expressed in the press and on TV not invariably clouded the main message and influenced our views. For some people these regular diets of information caused fear and anxiety about Covid-19 and worries about the future. The daily publication of deaths is a constant reminder to many that they are vulnerable and likely to succumb to the illness. The reduction in people seeking help for illnesses not related to Covid-19 shows the extent to which fear has gripped them. Fear of contracting Covid-19 lead many patients not to seek help for urgent and life-threatening conditions like heart attack and stroke.

For PoW's the biggest worry was how long they would remain

incarcerated. A second concern was whether they would survive the war. Death could occur unintentionally for example by bombardment of prisons by their own side, as part of collateral damage; a variety of 'friendly fire'. With Covid-19 also comes a large amount of uncertainty of how long lockdown would last and continuing worry about its consequences.

When historian Dr Clare Makepeace analysed the diaries of British PoW's during their incarceration she found that they did not despair of the state they were in. They also expressed no animosity towards their captors. Despite being bored they had hoped that their incarceration would soon end. Many of us too welcomed lockdown initially, thinking of it as an enforced holiday. But soon the monotony and realisation of the consequences of what had happened is likely to have caused anxiety, despair of the future, depression etc.

PoW's used their creativity to keep them occupied. For example they had amateur dramatics. These held them together and equally importantly reduced frictions among them. We have TV, Zoom, Skype etc. The National Theatre brought productions like Antony & Cleopatra and the Barber Shop Chronicles directly into our homes. Joe Wicks provided entertaining home exercise programs to keep us busy and fit at the same time. Like for the PoW's who had physical barbed wire to ensure continued incarceration, lockdown was a mental barbed wire which was there to prevent us escaping the confines of home. We needed to build a routine for coping with the isolation and boredom.

So is our lockdown 'home prison 'a gilded one compared to that of PoW's? We cannot compare the two, although our predicament in Covid-19 is also a risky one. Lockdown is a risk to health, career, finances etc.

Appearing on the Today program on television the psychiatrist, Sir Simon Wessely, comparing Covid-19 to war said that Covid-19 is different because unlike during the war, we cannot go to the cinema, shop freely, our children cannot go to school etc. In this respect the psychological consequences of lockdown are uncertain and as such we are in 'uncharted territory'.

Many POW's suffered depression, anger, fits of temper and claustrophobia.

The idea of a prison at home is one that is as unusual as it is difficult to accept. It also implies that 'home-prison' would be different things to different people, structurally and conceptually. Take the case of the man or the family living in a house in the country with a garden. For this person or family being at home would initially be welcome. After a fortnight or so it could, in many instances, be viewed as an inconvenience. The sense of space that the home gives helps to ameliorate the thought of it as a prison. You may have a separate room or an out-house where you could set up a home office or you may already have one. The concept of working from home may not be new but sustained working from home would require discipline. But this is possible and may turn out to be as productive as if one were in the office. Increased productivity in working from home has been often shown to be the case during lockdown. Many people working from home have realized that they are as productive as they were in an office and that the adjustment of working environment occurred without much effort. However, the availability of a home-office or even space at home to work may not be a luxury that everyone had. Or your work may not lend itself to working from home like a person working in manufacturing or in a car assembly plant or driving a bus, train or taxi. Such a person also, with a home and garden, could adapt to the new circumstances. However, in the latter case the lack of work is likely to eventually lead to monotony and frustration. But in both these situations what would be missing are the social interactions with others in the office, which is an integral part of the working day of many people. Establishing and maintaining links with colleagues is still possible and in several instances have continued unabated. The availability of means of communication has facilitated the continuation by virtual contact. Meetings on Skype, Zoom etc. have continued. For this reason the phrase 'social distancing' may not be appropriate. Social contacts can and have continued during lockdown. 'Physical distancing' may be a more accurate description for the separation of persons without necessarily diminishing social interaction.

Compare this situation with the millions who live in high-rise apartment blocks. Over twenty-five years ago I was introduced to the phrase 'human filing cabinets'. The significance of the phrase was lost on me at the time. Now with lockdown, quarantine and self-isolation, the phrase has assumed a frightening and less than benign meaning. Filing cabinets are structures where documents, objects etc are locked away from sight until when they are next needed. The drawers of the filing cabinet, not invariably, are slammed shut. Imagine if into each of the drawers of a filing cabinet was inserted a living human being and slammed shut! That is what happens in a block of apartments. The people in an apartment are the 'contents of the filing cabinet'. They are incarcerated behind the front door of their apartments and are asked to stay there during lockdown. They can go out only for food, medicine or a short period of exercise. And where do they exercise, other than in the communal spaces in the locality? Most modern apartments, fortunately, have a balcony which many occupants have transformed into a vibrant living area with plants, seating, lighting etc. This is an area of escapism for many in lockdown. Yet even the most well appointed apartment cannot provide relief from the boredom of lockdown which continues week after week behind the closed front door of the apartment. Prisons, penal institutions, correctional facilities etc are also 'human filing cabinets'.

Many apartments are tightly packed living spaces. The average flat or apartment in UK is 49 square metres. About 50% of Londoners live in apartments. Common complaints were that there was not enough room for furniture, not enough storage space and that occupants of apartments could not escape from noise generated by people in adjoining apartments. Even prior to lockdown, living in an apartment was stressful to many. Children may not have the space for play, for homework etc. even in normal circumstances.

The multiplicity of cramped domestic accommodation in the UK led the daily Telegraph to call it 'rabbit hutch Britain'. One may also call it 'human filing cabinet Britain'.

At the other extreme are those few persons with large houses and several acres of personal open space for whom lockdown may not have been a burden.

In 2007, Robert Gifford, a psychologist, wrote that children living in high-rise apartments have limited access to outdoor activity which may contribute to them having more behavioural problems. Another writer, Pearl Jephcott said in 1971 that living in a high-rise apartment is not satisfactory for a family with small children. It is also known that mothers living in apartments complained of loneliness and depression and the lack of space for their children to play. Taking these and other statements together it is not hard to appreciate the adverse effects of lockdown on the residents in high-rise apartment blocks. For children, who by their nature are usually adventurous, it is difficult to stay locked within the confines of an apartment. During lockdown, homes and especially apartments become emotional pressure cookers generating frustration, anger, resentment and depression. Covid-19 related lockdown was an additional pressure imposed on the already existing stress of living in cramped accommodation.

For children the value of going to school is probably greatest for those who come from apartment blocks. The release from their 'prison' may not be readily apparent to those who live in houses. For all of us, however, lockdown has brought home the important part played by school in the life of the children. School educates a child, keeps him occupied, helps develop social skills, counteracts boredom and sends him home tired at the end of the school day. What occurs in lockdown is probably little different to what parents go through during school holidays. But lockdown was sudden; there were no plans, no school homework etc. Some older children in higher grades at school are likely to occupy themselves with self-study. Keeping younger children occupied and entertained within the home and within an apartment is a challenge. How does one tell a child not to go out! How does one tell a child not to kick a ball or not to play?

Sudden cessation of a child's schooling is not only the interruption of education in the sense of learning in a classroom. It is also the absence of development of social skills – interaction with other children and teachers, learning and reciprocating common courtesies etc. While some parents may be able to provide a semblance of classroom education at home, this would still be challenging and fraught with frictions at home, the longer lockdown continued.

Inter-personal skills between adults at home would also be adversely affected and made worse by monotony and boredom. We have heard of the increase in domestic violence during lockdown.

Teenagers in lockdown would be easily bored. While they may find some solace on the internet this would come at price. Many parents have been trying to limit their children's time on the internet and have been trying to monitor the sites that their children access. This may not always be possible in lockdown and especially the longer it continues in its initial form. The effects of unrestricted internet access by children are largely unknown and society may count the cost in years to come.

Young persons who were planning to enter university or those who were awaiting graduation in 2020 are probably the most likely to be affected of the younger generation. As the Institute of Fiscal Studies notes, lockdown would affect employability and may contribute to reduced wages in those who are able to secure jobs. This is likely to adversely affect quality of life for many years going forwards.

Lockdown and information about Covid-19 has made many people fearful. Fear of catching the illness, fear of going to hospital and fear for loved ones. Fear generates anxiety which leads to depression which is made worse by the inability to meet with others. Daily reporting of the numbers of deaths and the total deaths make the sense of fear and panic worse. For some persons there is a pervading sense of impending doom. The elderly and those who are house bound are particularly susceptible to the feeling that life may be coming to an end.

Some of the things that affected PoW's were boredom and irritation with fellow prisoners, which was made worse by proximity to each other.

Irritation within the confines of our home 'prisons' leads not only to domestic violence but also to a whole range of minor irritations which we would normally put up with. As there is limited or no escapism in lockdown, these minor irritations and habits appear to be more frequent and could lead to frustration, and anger. Pent up anger causes arguments and violence - verbal or physical. Along with adult violence there is a risk of harm to children in a house. Child and adult safeguarding issues have increased during lockdown. Talking to some general medical practitioners it is clear that these are real issues which they encountered more in lockdown than before.

It is known that globally 30% of women experience physical or sexual violence during their life time. Often the perpetrator is a partner. Staying at home during lockdown, especially if the relationship with her partner was already an abusive one or even a strained one, increases the risk of violence for her. When the pandemic started in China, police in one province of Hubei reported a three times increased rate of domestic violence compared to the same period in 2019. In the UK the number of deaths from domestic violence in March-April 2020 was double the average of the previous ten years.

One police force in the UK made 400 arrests for domestic abuse during a fortnight of lockdown. The Boyzone singer Shane Lynch revealed that he moved out of the family home after arguing with his wife during lockdown. He claimed that he and wife were 'at each other's throats' due to lockdown. While this may be a high profile person whose case was reported in the press, it is likely this account reflects the many more relationships that have been strained during lockdown.

Research had shown that mental illness during lockdown had been higher than during the comparable time in 2019. Women with pre-school children appeared to have suffered considerable stress during lockdown. Some of those who were in employment prior to the pandemic suffered stress. This was related to uncertainty about returning to their previous jobs, being furloughed and appearing unemployed, reduction in income and trying to cope with new ways of working away from the usual workplace. People in lower income groups, who were black or of Asian origin suffered with more stress and in the 18-29 age group, researchers found increased anxiety, depression and thoughts of self-harm and death. These findings are in contrast with the effect of lockdown on people who were secure financially. This group benefitted from the greater amount of time with family, reduced stress and a better sense of feeling well.

However there was also evidence of feelings of relief during the pandemic and improvements in memory. Many people learned to cope well during the pandemic.

The Swiss physician Adolf Lukas Vischer wrote about 'Barbed Wire Disease". This was an account of the psychological harm to young people held in captivity in World War 1. He noted that those who had been in captivity for more than two years suffered restlessness, poor concentration and a loss of interest in life beyond the internment camp. The same problems were seen by British and Indian soldiers in Turkish captivity and in German PoW's held in the Isle of Man and on the British mainland. He concluded that what he observed was a human response to be held in camps behind barbed wire. The symptoms were solely related to duration of captivity and were independent of race, social class and religion. The

French described a condition called 'cafard' for what they interpreted as home-sickness in those in captivity.

In lockdown we have encountered a form of 'cafard' with separation from family. The various symptoms of 'barbed wire disease' have also been encountered, but in a much shorter time period than that observed during World War 1.

While there is likely to be a general increase in mental illness of varying degree as a result of lockdown, some are likely to be more severely affected. The provision of mental health services like counselling would be of help to many.

Loneliness has been a particular problem during lockdown. Prior to lockdown a survey showed that one in ten people felt lonely. But a few weeks after lockdown was imposed, almost one in four people complained of loneliness. Loneliness was more in those in the 18-24 year age group with over 40% saying that they felt lonely. In the short term, loneliness is not likely to be a problem. But the longer that lockdown continues and people are cut off from their usual contacts and from the ability to build new relationships etc., prolonged loneliness may lead to frustration, anxiety and depression.

Of the many psychological problems that arise in lockdown, alcoholism and addiction are common. Access to alcohol is easy and the temptation to consume more than what would have been average consumption, is great. Alcoholism is used by many to combat isolation and boredom. Being in the current 'home prison' there is also considerable worry about employment, finances, support for family etc. With anxiety and worry, many seek solace and escapism in alcohol. Excess alcohol consumption is not only a problem for those at home but also for those who work during lockdown. This is especially so for front line workers, who work long hours, deal with seriously ill patients, witness death more often than normal during their work. Alcohol would be seen as a relief from the stress of work. The same could be said of substance misuse. Some may experiment for the first time with cannabis or other drugs while those who are regular users of these drugs may increase consumption for the same reasons that alcohol does.

Anger is a common emotion to unusual events. Anger and frustration arises from concerns about careers, opportunities missed, relationships strained or fractured by lockdown etc.

Grief and bereavement following the loss of loved ones may be accompanied by depression. The lonely disposal of dead loved ones during lockdown has been a source for much grief in those left behind. The stories related by loved ones who could not be with or say a proper good bye to a beloved father, mother, grandparent etc made harrowing listening to many. One could not but be moved to tears for listening to these sad and poignant tales.

People with learning and /or intellectual disabilities are likely to experience heightened levels of stress and fear during lockdown. This is especially so if they have been through emotional or physical trauma in the past. Many of these persons enjoy and benefit for e.g. from even short journeys outside the home. Restriction of these simple activities is likely to be a concern to them; they may have difficulty understanding why they are confined at home and unable to go out as before. Add to this the likelihood of changes of carers that may be encountered and it is easy to see how confusion and frustration could follow. The need for carers, who are strangers, to wear personal protection equipment is likely to be upsetting or even frightening to those being cared for.

Many of the psychological consequences of lockdown may manifest later as post- traumatic stress disorder that is likely to need help for long periods.

Aiysha Malik of WHO believes that healthcare workers and children are some of those most affected by the Covid-19 crisis. Children are exposed to the same news as adults and are anxious, afraid for themselves, their immediate family and for their extended families. If a family member has or had Covid-19 or had died, this generates much greater fear of the illness together with grief. Parents, Malik believes, need to show resilience at this time to help guide their children through the crisis. If parents are seen as anxious, afraid or sad, these emotions are likely to be reflected in children.

A particularly unfortunate aspect of Covid-19 is stigmatisation. Stigmatisation of the person or even an entire family after one person had suffered the infection may cause all of them to be shunned by friends, neighbours and family. Fake news about Covid-19 may contribute to erroneous views about the disease that plays its part in people being marginalised or even ignored. One could become a social pariah. This would take a long time to recover from and may not be helped by continuation of the pandemic or the emergence of subsequent waves of the infection. The Cambridge English Dictionary defines a leper as a person 'who is strongly disliked and avoided by other people because of something bad that he or she has done' One hopes that society does not treat its fellow human beings as 'social lepers' during this pandemic.

Many would remember the stigmatisation, discrimination and abuse associated with HIV/ AIDS. It is worth recalling the words of Michel Sidibe, Executive Director of UNAIDS – 'Whenever AIDS has won, stigma, shame, distrust, discrimination and apathy was on its side. Every time AIDS has been defeated, it has been because of trust, openness, dialogue between individuals and communities, family support, human solidarity, and the human perseverance to find new paths and solutions'. These words are as relevant today as they have always been and are generally applicable to every aspect of human life.

We are advised always to avoid discrimination of any kind and at all times. But it is particularly important in the current climate to avoid discrimination not only because of a diagnosis of Covid-19 but also because of the ethnic origin of a person.

How have prisoners in 'real prisons' managed during lockdown? Prisoners are in a form of lockdown and are likely to be so for the duration of their sentences. Prisoners are literally and metaphorically within barbed wire. One would not be blamed for thinking that they would manage incarceration better because they are, apart from new inmates, somewhat accustomed to incarceration. But add to the prison environment the new need for physical distancing and the whole situation assumes a different form. Prisoners who may be two to a cell, needed to be separated. Additional temporary accommodation had been added outside the main blocks in some prisons so that social distancing could be maintained. As there are no toilet facilities in cells, some prisoners have had to use buckets in their cells. At other times there has had to be queuing to use the available toilets. Exercise was limited so that most prisoners spent almost 23 hours of each day locked up in their cells.

It was initially thought that there would be an explosion of Covid 19 in prisons. According to a paper by Miranda Davies of the Nuffield Trust titled "Covid-19: how is it impacting on prisoners' health?" PHE estimated that there was likely to be 77,800 cases of Covid-19 and 2,700 deaths from a prison population of around 81,000. Fortunately this scenario had not materialised and as of 15th June there were 502 positive cases of the virus among prisoners and 971 staff had also tested positive to the virus. There were 23 deaths among prisoners and 9 staff had died from the infection.

Self-harm rates were known to be increasing before the pandemic. There were 63,000 incidents of self-harm in 2019 and this was 14% greater than in 2018. What effects isolation due to Covid-19 would have was not known at the time of writing.

The provision of general medical services and the care of prisoner's physical health are also likely to be adversely affected. Initial triage would occur in the prisons but it is likely that there would be lesser numbers of prisoners conveyed to hospitals during lockdown.

The psychological consequences of Covid-19 and lockdown are likely to be around for a long time. As Hans Kluge, director of the European branch of the WHO said "This is not going to be a sprint, but a marathon,". He advised countries to prepare to deal with mental health problems of people.

Given the stresses that occur during lockdown it is not surprising that some have found it necessary to breach the guidance. Never in human history has almost the entire population of the world been imprisoned in their homes for the greater good of all. Never have governments across the world achieved such a very high degree of compliance with 'draconian' laws. The word 'coronavirus' was alien to many prior to the beginning of 2020. Never before have billions of people, all at much the same time, sought information on and educated themselves about a tiny organism, yet remained afraid of and yearned for escape from it.

Lockdown fatigue is a feeling of tiredness and exhaustion despite being less active. It probably linked to the loss of a routine to daily life. Humans are creatures of habit and live through a series of personal algorithms each day. The loss or disruptions of the sequential series of acts during the day contributes to boredom and lethargy. At the same time there is an increased alertness and worry coupled with fear about infection and the need to take preventive measures like social distancing and hand- washing. Poor sleep is not uncommon. The heightened alertness in some people is similar to that experienced during post-traumatic stress disorder (PTSD).

Diverting boredom to creativity is a common form of 'productive escapism'. Thank goodness for the internet. Humanity can now engage in all types of virtual activities. Take the case of 15 year old Jaden Ashman in 2019, before lockdown was even on the horizon. He shared the second prize of £1.8 million with his partner Dave Jong at the 2019 gaming championships in the Arthur Ashe Stadium in New York. Over forty million people had tried to qualify for the championships. Eventually there were 100 finalists from 30 countries. The winner of the three million dollar first prize was a 16 year old boy from Pennsylvania. It therefore seems that the time your teenager spends on the internet may not always be bad and that it has it upsides.

Jaden's mother was apparently not pleased with him spending time gaming and not doing his homework. But he was productive! .

Another useful example is that of 17 year old Avi Schiffmann from Seattle who had been tracking coronavirus since December 2019. He finally devised a Covid-19 tracker in his bedroom – ncov2019.live. He is pleased that he has 'created something that helps millions of people around the world'. He hoped other teenagers also would 'create cool stuff'.

It is said that there is no system of education yet devised that can hold back someone driven to achieve. To some people lockdown is not a disadvantage that cannot be overcome. Daily routine may be exchanged for investment in things that are productive. Lockdown is an opportunity to some.

According to Stephen Reicher from St.Andrew's University in Scotland, lockdown not only has psychological effects but also physical effects on people. It is bad for your health and can increase the risk of death by up to 30%. It can have as bad an impact on a person as smoking or obesity. It can be as damaging to health as smoking 15 cigarettes a day.

Whatever negative aspects there were as a result of lockdown it is an inescapable fact that many people were happy and contended in lockdown. How could this be when life has almost instantaneously been turned upside down? Human beings are resilient even in the most adverse conditions. This is due to the phenomenon of 'hedonic adaptation', which is the tendency of humans to somewhat quickly return to their previous state of happiness or unhappiness following positive or negative events in life. This adaptation is best seen in people who have unfortunately encountered severe adverse events in life. Take for example those who suffer the locked-in syndrome. This happens after a stroke which affects the brainstem, where most of the control centres of the body are. After a period of unconsciousness the person recovers to a completely paralysed state unable to move any of the limbs. They cannot talk but are able to see, hear and have some eye movements. They are able to think rationally and their intelligence is unaffected. This leaves the person with the ability to communicate with the outside world only with their eyes or what is left of their cheek movements. These limited retained movements are deployed to control a computer by means of a suitably connected stick or by other communication devices. Steven Laureys and his colleagues from the Neurology Department and Cyclotron Research Centre, University of Liège, Belgium wrote that most of these patients, when questioned, said that they were happy. More importantly, they wrote that these persons 'should not be denied the right to live - and to live with dignity'. So it is that many, if not the majority of people coped very well during lockdown.

Could we have weathered the storm of Covid-19 without lockdown? It is felt that lockdown should have been imposed earlier than it was on 23rd of March. The justification for lockdown is proven if there are other general or localized waves of the infection following release from it. We have been in a similar situation before. In 1938 it was thought that a coordinated air raid could kill 50,000 and injure 300,000 more people. Such a scale of injuries and death would have been an enormous psychological blow to public morale. At the same time, such a cataclysmic event would have been an intolerable burden on the health services of the time. A succession of such air raids would have incapacitated the country. The thought of air raids and those air raids that occurred spread fear and panic among the population. Much the same has happened with Covid-19 in 2020. In 1938 however Wilfred Trotter, a neurosurgeon of the time, wrote that 'the common people- as always, the moral backbone of the country, – resisted and at length threw it off'.

Many have questioned the need for lockdown. Initially the government said it was to 'Save the NHS'. But Lord Sumption a judge of the Supreme Court in the UK, asked whether the NHS needed to be protected when it is there to protect the public. But by invoking lockdown, use of NHS facilities diminished so much so that people's lives continued to be at risk form delayed diagnosis and treatment of cancer, heart attacks etc. Fear of using the NHS from fear of contracting Covid-19 in hospitals and not from an altruistic desire to save the NHS led to the NHS having spare capacity. Therefore there was no real need for use of the Nightingale Hospitals. The benefit of lockdown was initially to help retain capacity in the NHS. This would have helped the NHS to deal with any large scale surge in demand for treatment of Covid-19 patients, especially the need for ventilation of those who are seriously ill from it. The history of epidemics and pandemics of the past and the large numbers of deaths that had occurred may have influenced politicians in their decisions. Scientific advisers can use information from the past but can only surmise what could happen in the future. Models of probable numbers of deaths from Covid-19 are based on many variables, any one or more of which could widely skew the predicted numbers of deaths. Led by scientific advice the ultimate decision, as in war, has to be a political one. Therefore lockdown came into being for the benefit of all of us.

C. S. Lewis wrote 'of all tyrannies, a tyranny sincerely exercised for the good of its victims may be the most oppressive'. Lockdown was not an exercise in benevolent tyranny; there was a genuine need for it, based on the evidence of history and the modelling of scientists and mathematicians. The numbers of possible deaths of 250,000 may have been a worst case estimate but decision makers may have been cognizant of the many millions who died in the Spanish flu of 1918 and in the plague of the 14th century.

As Donna Barbisch wrote in 2015, lockdown is a legally enforceable police power applied as a public health measure. Lockdown and quarantine have their basis in international Law. The International Health Regulations of the WHO were reiterated in 2005 as a means of containing infection and preventing its spread across international boundaries. However it is up to each country or jurisdiction to apply quarantine and lockdown as it sees most appropriate in the circumstances.

To have left people to make an informed choice on how they acted, when given the information about Covid-19, would have been dangerous. Individual choice and autonomy of the person would have placed many persons at risk and may have made real the worse case estimates of deaths. Doing nothing was not an option. We see the emergence of increasing cases of covid-19 and deaths in Sweden, which did not enforce a lockdown.

Donna Barbisch and her colleagues wrote that politicians need to be guided by evidence when applying quarantine and they must be influenced by the likelihood of improved outcomes when suspension of civil liberties is being considered. Any such restrictive measures should also be capable of implementation. The latter has been largely achieved by the authorities. As regards the former, it is near impossible to predict the possible outcomes, especially of lockdown. Warfare of any kind is unpredictable in its outcome. Lockdown and quarantine while necessary, would be accepted by the majority, grudgingly complied with by many and ignored by a few. Daisy Fancourt and colleague wrote in May 2020 that only 40% of young people in their survey complied with guidelines. Anxiety and depression was above average with the former being worse in the young, in those with children and in those with pre-existing mental health conditions.

However, those who oppose lockdown need to ask how they choose to protect themselves and others from Covid-19. The evolving nature of the pandemic, our limited knowledge about the virus and the lack of effective treatment or vaccine would have made the task of any government a difficult one. Government would be held to account if it was seen to have over-reacted by imposing a lockdown or to have under-reacted, if there was an increasing death toll and a second and successive waves of the infection. Jeffrey M. Drazen, Rupa Kanapathipillai and colleagues wrote in the New England Journal of Medicine in 2015 about Ebola that 'we should be guided by the science…'And that is what was needed with Covid-19, although evidence was initially lacking and our knowledge base about the infection is as changing as it is increasing.

However, all countries did not apply lockdown in the same manner. Sweden stands out as how one country chose to interpret International Health regulations. Sweden's population generally accepted what its government advises without the need for a legally enforced lockdown. The usual advice regarding keeping a safe distance from others, hand- washing, working from home etc are followed by the Swedes without the need for legislation. As a population which regularly follows the advice of its government, it is easy for accepted practice to take place without the need to enforce it. This is not a case of ignoring the science or an example in the demonstration of liberty. But as the Prime Minister of Sweden, Stefan Löfven, said it is looking at the disease as a long term event and playing to contain the total number of deaths over a longer period. Time will tell if the Swedish experiment is right. But even there, the public have accepted the advice to be safe and have complied with it.

It appears reasonable to think of Covid-19 as a long term pandemic with which the public in many countries would have to contend with. In the middle of August one encountered a spike in the illness in several countries in Europe. Numbers of cases per million of the population was 35 in France, 44 in the Netherlands and 80 in Malta. Even New Zealand and Australia were dealing with re-appearance of cases of Covid-19. Therefore the approach of Sweden may yet turn to be a correct one.

'Barbed wire disease' 2020.

o0:0o

COLLATERAL DAMAGE

While lockdown is a necessity there are down sides to it which affects individuals and society at large. Apart from the personal effects of incarceration, economic consequences etc there are personal health problems unrelated to Covid-19 which are exacerbated or arise anew during lockdown.

Early on in lockdown the European Society of Cardiology showed that there was nearly a 75% reduction in emergency attendances and admission for symptoms of heart attacks. This was seen across countries in Europe. This finding does not imply that Covid-19 is somehow benevolent and protective to the heart. Nothing could be further than this impression. There is no evidence that the infection adversely affects the heart in the same way that it causes inflammation in and damages our lungs. On the other hand Covid-19 has instilled fear in all of us. The fear of attending hospital for illnesses that are serious and that could be fatal in themselves, but which have nothing to do with Covid-19, has prevented people from seeking medical help. If one has chest pain, one is advised by the British Heart Foundation to seek help early, if only to exclude a heart attack. Many people with chest pain could go on to have a heart attack. Many of these patients would be transferred to cardiac (heart) centres and have a stent inserted or even heart bypass surgery. This is life saving work. The consequences of not seeking help for chest pain is that those whose pain is due to a heart attack are at a great risk of sudden death and later problems like heart failure, if they survive the initial event. Seeking help later, after a heart attack, is more difficult to manage. If the heart does not pump as well as it did before a heart attack one get heart failure. This is more difficult to manage and carries a risk of earlier death.

Dr Sonya Babu-Narayan, associate medical director of the British Heart Foundation said that in June 2020 there were 28,000 patients awaiting heart procedures which had been postponed during lockdown.

Cancer Research UK said that about 2300 cancers were not being diagnosed every week during the lockdown. This means that 2300 patients with cancer are having their diagnosis of it missed or delayed. Patients in the UK are usually referred by their general medical practitioners (GP's) using the 2 week-wait referral pathway. This ensures that patients with possible cancer are seen in the NHS by a relevant specialist within 2 weeks of being referred by their GP. We know that these referrals are taking place because they have not ceased. At the onset of lockdown it was decided that referral for suspected cancer would continue as an essential service. This service, therefore, did not cease in lockdown. If these referrals are not happening to the same extent that they were happening before lockdown, it means that some patients may either be ignoring their symptoms or are postponing consulting with their GP's. In April 2020, data showed that urgent cancer referral by general practitioners was 60% less than at the same time in 2019. The only logical explanation for this is that patients are afraid of consulting their GP's for fear of being referred to hospitals. With hospitals seeing and treating patients with Covid-19, hospitals are perceived by the public to be danger areas. Hospitals are to be avoided at any cost. It was estimated that delays in diagnosis and treatment could eventually lead to 7000 excess deaths. This figure was arrived at by modeling which also showed that in a worst case scenario there could be as much as 35,000 excess cancer deaths.

Unfortunately the cost incurred here is to personal health. Sadly some, if not many, of these patients may be in need of urgent medical treatment for their symptoms like increasing bleeding from the back passage or an enlarging ulcer on the skin. Diagnosis of cancer, when eventually made, would be at a more advanced stage than if patients were seen earlier. Linked to this is the fact that treatment of advanced cancer is more complex than at the outset of the disease when it is likely to have been of a lower grade of cancer. Early operation in some cases is curative. This means that for all intents and purposes the patient is cured of the cancer. Some patients may reach the stage where the delay in seeking medical help has made the cancer inoperable. Many patients with cancer have an operation followed by radiotherapy and/ or chemotherapy. This treatment plan is to make the patient free of cancer, as far as possible. The opportunity to achieve this aim in treatment of a patient with cancer would be lost when the patient presents late.

Cancer Research UK said that the impact of COVID-19 on cancer patients is "devastating". There has been a 60% reduction in referrals for cancer compared to a similar time in 2019. This, according to Cancer Research UK, translates into several thousands of patients needing 'vital care'.

The Teenage Cancer Trust has 28 specialist cancer units across the UK which treats 13 to 24 year olds who are diagnosed with cancer. The Trust has been collecting informal data which showed that referrals for cancer in this age group had fallen in April and May 2020. Director of the Teenage Cancer Trust, Dr Louise Soanes, said: "We know that seven young people every day get diagnosed with cancer but many of our nurses are reporting back to us that in their area, they are seeing reductions. Some haven't had any new cases referred in some weeks whilst others have gone from having three a week to one or two." Another aspect of the impact of Covid-19 has been the delay or cancellation of operations and other treatments for cancers in this age group. This undoubtedly caused a lot of anxiety among teenagers and young persons. When operation or other treatments took place, it was with staff using personal protective equipment. The lack of direct face-to-face contact with staff these young persons and children had got accustomed to caused worry and fear. Also being confined in a room without contact with others was to some a cause for depression.

Many in the public do not realize that hospitals have dedicated Covid-19 areas. The rest of the hospital is technically free of Covid-19 and allows for treatment of other medical conditions. The NHS is trying to manage this worry by setting up Covid-free cancer hubs. Novel ways of delivering care are being used to help provide much needed, life-saving cancer care to patients. Some hospital trusts have provided 'chemotherapy buses'. These vehicles reach out to patients in their communities and provide chemotherapy without exposure to a hospital environment. Each bus is fully equipped to deliver chemotherapy and can hold four patients at a time, complying with physical distancing rules. Some patients are having their chemotherapy at home by specially trained staff, again avoiding the need to visit a hospital. These methods of delivery of care help to allay patient's fears while ensuring that continuity of care is maintained.

A survey found that a fifth of patients did not see their General Practitioners (GP) during lockdown because of worries about Covid-19 or that they did not want to burden the NHS. Forty percent of those surveyed said that they worry about going to hospital. One in ten people said they could not get a dental appointment with 50% of respondents saying they were in pain. Women are more worried and cautions about seeking medical help than men.

The National Health Service (NHS) in the UK provides screening services for the population in UK. A range of medical conditions are screened for in accordance with accepted principles for screening. In lockdown the NHS screening programs for cervical, breast and bowel cancers had been temporarily suspended. This added to another group of cancers which would be missed or where the early diagnosis would have been delayed. The people who are invited for screening are those who do not have symptoms and but who could have early cancers. These are called pre-symptomatic cancers; cancers long before symptoms appear. This is an important group of patients with cancer where early diagnosis and treatment is likely to make a vital difference to their health and length and quality of life. When these cancers are eventually detected after lockdown has been eased, they are likely, in some cases, to be in a later stage of the disease. Or some of these cancers which did not cause symptoms may reach a stage at which they cause symptoms. They could only cause symptoms if the cancer has progressed from the stage at which it was pre-symptomatic. In other words the cancer is now in a more advanced stage than had it been detected by screening and before the onset of symptoms. About 2.4 million people are waiting for cancer screening tests. Four hundred cancers are picked up each week by screening. This is the equivalent to a potential of 23,000 cancers not being diagnosed during lockdown.

In June it was reported that since the onset of lockdown 12,750 (40%) fewer patients have undergone cancer surgery, 6000 (30%) fewer have received chemotherapy and 2800 (10%) fewer have had radiotherapy for their cancers.

The reduction in diagnoses of cancer combined with the reduced availability of operative surgery, radiotherapy etc points to a near epidemic of cancer that is awaiting the NHS. The surge in cancers is likely to contribute to as many or more premature deaths than does Covid-19. The total deaths from non-Covid health problems are likely to exceed Covid-19 deaths by a significant magnitude. This is why Professor Carol Sikora, a specialist in cancer care, has called for a plan to deal with the crisis in care that is likely to confront the UK in the post-Covid period. He makes a plea that the NHS avoids going along in a 'business as usual' mode. He makes a cogent case for movement away from surgery and towards precision methods of radiotherapy and chemotherapy using drugs.

The Covid-19 pandemic has shown the need to keep cancer units free of Covid-19. This means that they need to be as far as possible 'structurally separate' from the rest of the hospital. Also staff need to be free of the infection. The phrase 'structurally safe' does not only or always mean a separate building. There needs to be a separate part of the hospital or a separate building in the hospital campus that is dedicated to cancer care; a form of medical 'Chinese wall'. Only staff who would be Covid-free would enter and leave the cancer unit and would not have dealings with or be deployed to other parts of the hospital or the NHS. Testing of staff is crucial and Prof Sikora cites the testing regime in the Premier League of football as an example that may be followed. Here players are tested regularly and those who have the infection are kept away for the mandatory period before they are allowed to return to the club, training facilities etc.

Another important feature that Prof. Sikora speaks of is the need to monitor positive biopsy numbers that come from pathology laboratories. These laboratories test specimens for cancer. A regular count of positive cancer tests on biopsy would give a useful indication of the increase in diagnosis and of the 'surge' of cancer. While the nation and the NHS nervously waits for a second spike in Covid-19, they appear to be blinded to the obvious surge in cancer and other serious conditions like cardiovascular disease. If we are 'all in this together' as regards Covid-19, then we are much the same with other aspects of healthcare, especially with cancer and heart disease. Suffering and death from non-Covid medical causes may finally surpass Covid-19. This is an important aspect to think about as the nation embarks on release from lockdown. The NHS and its staff need to look at imaginative ways of working to surmount what is likely to be a 'medical tsunami'. But it can be done.

The NHS Confederation is a body that represents all sectors of health and social care in England and Wales. It was formerly the National Association of Health Authorities and Trusts. Today it represents social care, hospital and community services, ambulance trusts and clinical commissioning groups which oversee primary care. The NHS Confederation is therefore an organization that speaks for the whole of the NHS. NHS Confederation is concerned about waiting lists for treatment, in the NHS. Waiting lists in the NHS stood at 4.2 million before the onset of the Covid-19 crisis. Since the crisis, the Confederation has warned of a big increase in waiting lists of patients awaiting treatment by the NHS and for other aspects of care. It is projected that the waiting list could increase to 10 million by the end of the year. The challenge for the NHS and the government is how this backlog would be managed, especially with social distancing that needs to take place and therefore the logistics of providing safe care. Inevitably the increased concerns about prevention of infection and the changes in working that would be needed is likely to severely slow down the rate at which care can be provided. This is likely to reduce the numbers of patients who could be treated safely. All of the time, however, numbers of people would continue to be added to waiting lists, as they increasingly use the NHS.

The UK is not alone in seeing the disruption to its usual health services during the Covid-19 pandemic. Dr Rosa Giuliani, director of public policy at the European Society of Medical Oncology said that the fallout from the Covid-19 will continue for the near future, at the least. The WHO published on 1st June its document 'Rapid assessment of service delivery for NCDs during the COVID-19 pandemic'. Here the WHO claimed that there is likely to be a long-term upsurge in deaths from non-communicable diseases (NCD's). The progress made worldwide in improving health and survival from NCDS has gradually gone down since 2010. The more severe the transmission phase of Covid-19 the greater is the disruption to services for the care of people with NCD's. For e.g. in 41% of countries surveyed cancer services were disrupted, while in 24% there was disruption in services for cardiovascular emergencies. WHO sated that 'the world is at a critical juncture'. This resonates with the views of Prof. Sikora in respect of services in the UK. The adverse effects of Covid-19 on other life-saving healthcare services, which are unconnected with the health effects of the pandemic, are likely to overtake that of the pandemic.

Dr.Giuliani discussed the difficult conversations that doctors have had and continue to have with patients. At the outset of the pandemic patients were told not to come to hospital for the sake of their health. Some cancer patients may have been surprised or even dismayed that their life-saving treatment was likely to be delayed or even not provided. Others had probably already made the decision not to attend hospital appointments for their own safety. Following release from lockdown and with the gradual resumption of services, doctors were advising patients to return to hospital for continuing their treatment and care. To convince vulnerable people to come back into the hospital environment is challenging, to say the least.

An important area that has been adversely affected by lockdown is the care of women in pregnancy. Across the whole duration of pregnancy, labour and in the post-natal period, social distancing and the need for patients and carers to remain safe has imposed various restrictions on access to maternity services. Women are reluctant to attend their GP's and midwives for antenatal care or these are conducted on the phone or through the medium of video calls. Various antenatal scans may have been delayed or even cancelled. Even when pregnant women attended these appointments the usual presence of a partner was not permitted during Covid-19. Ultrasound scans in pregnancy are vital for the detection of foetal abnormality, checking the baby' growth etc. The isolation felt by mothers following discharge from hospital should not be under-estimated. This is a challenging time for most, but especially for a first –time mother. For those with children, the need to care for the newborn while caring for other children becomes difficult, with no or only limited access to family and friends.

It remains important for health services of all kinds to be delivered while being mindful of patient and personnel safety. Health services need to adapt and continue with innovation in the way services are delivered.

If Covid-19 tested the ability of the NHS to protect the public from the infection while protecting itself, it has yet to rise to the challenge of its ultimate legacy during the pandemic. The lasting effects on the NHS, on those who work in it and on the health of the nation may be the most important words written about the effect of the pandemic on the NHS.

Human interaction with others creates society and binds a community providing social cohesion and preventing 'social sliding'. Social cohesion is a peculiar concept. We don't always think of it. But we contribute to it and participate in it without stopping for a moment to think about it. If society did not have unwritten rules by which people abide and which bind people together it would disintegrate in a 'social slide'. The glue that binds people together is not determined by colour, creed, religious belief, sexual preferences etc. The 'social glue' cannot be made by laws, Equality and Diversity legislation etc. It is the inherent feeling of individuals to belong to groups, live among others and to contribute to the greater good while respecting man-made laws and individual privacy. The majority of people comply with the laws of the land even if some may disagree with some of the laws. When we disagree we give voice to it in discussion, debate, elections etc. But most people go with the majority view of what is perceived in the situation and at the time, to be the best course to follow. The stronger the bonds the more cohesive and tolerant the society is. Everyone 'plays by the rules'. For e.g. the humanitarianism demonstrated in Britain following the Boxing Day tsunami of 2004 that devastated Asia, showed the fundamental need to help, among the vast majority of people. This led to a speedy response as judged by the amount of funds raised in the UK to help those who were affected by the tsunami. The need to help at times of need is one of the most important but silent catalysts that binds people together and contributes to the concept of 'being human'. Irrespective of the size of a person's contribution, the recognition of the immense need of other people at that time and the overwhelming desire to help demonstrated the bonds that bind people together. There is much more that unites people than ever has separated them.

At no time in recent history has social cohesion and social capital been put to the test than they have during the pandemic and in lockdown. The phrase 'social distancing' would ideally be replaced with 'physical distancing' as has been suggested by some writers. We have not reduced our social interactions with our friends, family, neighbours etc. We have continued our many and varied associations as far as they are possible as before, but keeping a healthy physical distance to prevent spread of infection. There was only a physical change due to the necessities of the time; it was not a social change. The cohesion that holds our societies together have continued irrespective of lockdown. How then can this cohesion be fractured during or because of lockdown? The single most important determinant of a breakdown in social cohesion is a breach of trust. The acts of some opinion formers and leaders in not abiding by the rules that have been set out for the benefit of all, causes a fissure and creates a feeling of 'them' and an 'us'.

The 'Black Lives Matter' protests, which coincided with Covid-19, are another example where a crack had developed in society. The Black Lives Matter (BLM) protests are important to highlight the issues that sections of the population feel strongly about. It is only right that a democracy, like the UK, gives space for this voice to be heard. However we are in the midst of a pandemic and, as has been said by the scientific community, this is a 'dangerous time'. We are gradually coming out of lockdown while warily keeping an eye on the R figure of infectivity of the virus. Release from lockdown may lead to another spike in infections and therefore a rise in the numbers who die from Covid-19. But people need to speak, they need to protest, their voices need to be heard.

Physical distancing is a vital part of containing the spread of infection. One heard the cries of the protestors who attended the BLM rallies. To some of them the BLM issue is a more potent 'virus' than Covid-19, it is as bad or even a worse than the pandemic. But by ignoring physical distancing during the rallies, the protesters were placing themselves and their communities at considerable risk. They were also placing everyone else at risk. It is as if to say that at that moment only black lives mattered. Was this a safe position to assume? And do not other lives matter, as obviously they do during the pandemic and in lockdown.

Irrespective of the merits of the case, the BLM rallies have been a flagrant breach of the lockdown regulations. If one sector of the population is permitted to break the rules en mass, how could they be enforced on others? The same could be said of the Extinction Rebellion protests in London. More hazardous are local lockdowns, if these were used. Some community leaders have expressed the view that these would be difficult to enforce in some areas for e.g. in the northwest of England. This is especially so if less affluent areas are placed in local lockdowns while more affluent areas with better housing and generally better quality of life are unaffected. One could then see a social divide appearing which would be a threat to social unity. This is a foundation for civil riots.

Community leaders have warned of the need for law enforcement agencies to build bridges with their local communities. This is best done with visible, yet sensible, policing together with effective heath promotion on the ground, in the areas affected by lockdown.

While talking about physical effects we should not forget the mental and psychological impact that lockdown has on people. Suddenly a massive change was imposed on all our lives by lockdown. We had to stay at home except for a few excursions outside. We were confined to the limited space of our homes and asked to spend the rest of the time there. The duration of this incarceration was uncertain. We were not used to this, however much we loved our homes. It was therefore inevitable that the stress of staying 'permanently indoors' would eventually tell on people, some being more affected than others. Those with existing mental health issues were likely to suffer a worsening of their condition. With limited access to mental health support staff, key workers and to outpatient appointments they now had to cope on their own, as best they could.

Anxiety and depression in those without previous mental health problems have also risen. These are often due to isolation, loss of job or the threat of it, reduced income and domestic and financial pressure. Living all the time with family or partners without the ability to go out is stressful. The feelings of entrapment in loneliness lead to insecurity and a loss of hope.

The elderly are particular prone to depression. Some of them lead lonely lives. Now with lockdown the little contact they had with friends and family were severely curtailed. The added elements of fear of the virus and the news of loss of loved ones, friends etc to the virus, lead to an increase in anxiety and worry.

Loneliness is not only a problem for the elderly. Before lockdown one in six young persons aged between 18 and 24 years said that they felt lonely. This figure had risen to 45% in lockdown. With continuing loneliness comes the risk of anxiety, depression and other mental health issues. Fears about continuing education, employment prospects and the future contributed to anxiety in lockdown.

Eugenio Proto from the University of Glasgow and Climent

Quintana-Domeque from the University of Exeter looked at the effects of Covid-19 on the mental health of people. Their findings confirm what was already known; there has been a general deterioration in mental health across the population in the UK. However detailed analysis revealed some interesting facts. Especially, the deterioration in the mental health of men was greater in the BAME population than in comparable British white men. This ethnic difference was not seen for women where the worsening of mental health during the pandemic was the same in both ethnic groups. When they looked at male BAME individuals it was found that the worsening of mental health was highest in Indian, Pakistani and Bangladesh men. It is obvious that further research is needed to find out the reasons for these ethnic differences. In conclusion BAME individuals are not only at greater risk from Covid-19 but also lockdown has a greater effect on the mental health of BAME men.

The changes in the way bereavements are dealt with during lockdown are a particular source of sadness to all. A loved one is often alone in hospital or in a care home with no contact with family and loved ones. Or there is only remote contact through digital media or through a window pane or transparent screen. The inability to be close to, touch, hear loved ones is a particularly distressing aspect of bereavement during the crisis. All these add to extended grief and in some cases to depression. The bereaved person often lives long in the minds of those who are left behind. I am aware of a few cases where compassionate nursing staff had, within safe limits, permitted family to approach and see a loved one who is at the end of life. These instances must have been sources of great comfort amidst the overwhelming grief of the moment.

Alcohol consumption during lockdown was a particular issue with some countries banning the sale of alcohol for certain periods. Isolation at home increases the risk of excessive alcohol consumption and drug use. These were likely to lead to domestic abuse. Those partners who had been in an abusive relationship were in greater danger of repeated violence. And to the victim the ability to escape from or contact sources of help or even to just have a conversation with a friend was virtually impossible and fraught with danger and the risk of more violence. It is no surprise that homicide rates have gone up during lockdown.

Refuge, which is the UK's largest domestic abuse charity, said that in the first two weeks of lockdown calls to its helpline rose by 25 per cent. In the same period calls to the National Domestic Abuse Helpline also increased by 25 per cent. In the same period hits to www.nationaldahelpline.org.uk, the national domestic abuse website, increased by 150 per cent. The Metropolitan Police reported that on average 100 people each day were arrested for domestic violence offences during the lockdown. These figures reflect the extent of despair and suffering of some who have been incarcerated at home. And the available figures for domestic violence during lockdown may not give a true picture of the extent of the problem.

The story of one victim, reproduced from a newspaper is described here.

Nicola (not her real name) who has a daughter had reached the end of her tether in her relationship with her partner, even before lockdown was introduced. She was planning to leave her partner when lockdown came into effect. She could not return to her mother, who was herself ill.

'I felt like I was trapped before quarantine happened, but now everything is a hundred times more intense....I feel guilty for not being stronger sooner. I'm exhausted and I just want a way out....I had prepared to leave my boyfriend and organised to go and stay with my mum, but then when the restriction came in, I wasn't able to travel and with my mum's already poor health, I couldn't risk going there'.

This is a tale of a not uncommon abusive relationship which had been made worse by lockdown.

Alarming figures show that by 31st of May calls to the National Domestic Abuse Helpline had increased by 66% while access to its website increased by a staggering 950 per cent.

In the first three weeks of lockdown there had been at least 16 suspected domestic abuse killings in the UK. Dame Vera Baird, the Victims Commissioner for England and Wales provided this information to a group of MP's. 'We usually say there are two a week that looks to me like five a week, that's the size of this crisis.' Said Dame Baird. This is the highest number of women killed by men in three weeks in the last eleven years.

Dame Vera Baird said that she did not believe that the coronavirus creates violent men. It is just that abuse is common and that lockdown was a trigger or an excuse for greater violence. This is made worse by the sense of entrapment that women feel and not being able to access outside sources of support and help. They are effectively cut off from the outside world with the abuser having total control.

Counting Dead Women is a project, founded by Karen Ingala Smith that records the killing of women by men in the UK. She says that one of the infuriating things for an abuser is to lose control over his victim. She thinks that release from lockdown may be a critical time for victims as the abuser may fear losing control. This may cause them to kill their victims.

Suicide is also on the increase during lockdown. Pensioners and those who are lonely are particularly at risk of suicide. Dr Amanda Thompsell, who is chair of the Faculty of Old Age Psychiatry, said that the elderly 'have been particularly hit by social isolation. They have been cut off from families, their routines disrupted and they had suffered disproportionately more bereavements of relatives and friends whose funerals they could not attend due to health risks'. One hospital trust has seen as many suicide attempts in the past two months as they had seen in the whole of the past year. Dr Janine Gronewold, a psychologist, said that suicides have increased worldwide due to the coronavirus. Fear has been the biggest trigger in most suicides.

A not uncommon form of abuse is that perpetrated by children and adolescents on their parents – children and adolescent parent violence (C/APV). A report by Rachel Condry, Professor of Criminology in the University of Oxford and Dr. Caroline Law, senior lecturer in Criminology in the University of Manchester describes the increase in C/APV during lockdown. This is not a new phenomenon that emerged during lockdown. C/APV had been happening before. However lockdown has increased the frequency of violence; police reported that they had encountered about 400 cases of C/APV. In most instances violent children have themselves been in receipt of violence and had safeguarding concerns. Unfortunately during lockdown, safeguarding services have reduced and have of necessity been delivered remotely. Parents who are in receipt of violence have often not reported events to the police for fear of giving children a criminal record or placing them at risk of Covid-19 following arrest. As such, many cases of C/APV have gone unreported. Some of the violence directed towards parents has been severe, as described by one mother whose son 'beat me so badly that if the police did not come when they did, I would not be alive'.

Perhaps the most significant collateral damage from lockdown is the effect on schoolchildren who have not been to school for several months. And there is continuing disagreement whether children are safe to return to school. The Childhood Trust has written about the educational attainment gap that existed before Covid-19 and lockdown. This gap is related to 'class' and economic status. For example research has shown that children who are entitled to free school meals have lower educational attainment. Children from middle and higher income groups are more likely to have access to and to pursue online learning compared to children from working class families. And families from the former two groups tend to assist their children more with their education. The Chartered College of Teaching produced a report - 'Education in times of crisis: The potential implications of school closures for teachers and students'. The report cited research to describe that 'summer learning loss' is greater in children from lower income families and these effects are greater in older children than in younger children. The report also referred to the greater adverse effect that school closures have on children with mental health issues.

The education of generations of children is likely to be affected the longer lockdown continues. When these children become adults their employability and life opportunities are likely to be adversely affected. This in turn works through into poor life choices, poor health and the risk of early mortality. There is therefore a moral imperative that children return to school and do so at the earliest opportunity. This does not imply that safety in relation to second or subsequent spikes of the pandemic need to be ignored. On the contrary novel ways of school attendance, teaching and learning are needed. We saw that in Germany towards the end of August there was a surge in cases in about 36 schools within a fortnight of them re-opening. The national rate of coronavirus was 11.5 new cases per 100,000 people. While this was low compared to France (18 per 100,000 people) and Spain (86 per 100,000 people) the authorities were concerned sufficiently to take necessary action. Angela Merkel, the German Chancellor, blamed returning travellers from Turkey and the Balkan countries and private parties for the rise in cases. In North Rhine-Westphalia teachers and pupils were compelled to wear face masks while in France children over the age of 11 years returning to school in September would have to wear face masks. Bickering between various stakeholders does little to reassure parents and children that their interests are given the urgent attention that they so rightly deserve.

The effect on the economy of the UK has been alarming. In April 2020 the economy shrunk by 20.4% and the country is in recession. Compare this figure with the decline of 5.8% in March and 0.2% in February. UK borrowing in March 2020 was £3.9bn more than in March 2019; and this was before coronavirus and the lockdown that followed it. Even as early as April 2020 it was obvious that the economic impact of lockdown was likely to be quite severe. The combination of markedly reduced retail sales and other economic activity together with a record number of people claiming benefit showed that the economy was contracting and that the fiscal deficit was increasing. As long as lockdown continued and with reduced economic activity, tax receipts were also likely to fall considerably. The Office of National Statistics said that retail sales in March reduced by 5% compared to February 2020. This was with only an 8-day period of lockdown and was due to closure of shops that did not sell essential items like food. This fall was the biggest monthly fall in retail sales in thirty years. The only saving grace was the increase in retail activity in supermarkets with sales of food and related items. In fact supermarkets recorded an increase in trading due, no doubt, to panic buying by shoppers and to hoarding.

In the end of May, the Chancellor announced that the furlough scheme would end in October 2020. The scheme has been a lifeline to many employees; it has supported about 8.4 million workers. However many people have lost their jobs and others who are on furlough are uncertain as to whether they would have a job to return to. To meet the requirements of furlough and to support the economy, government borrowing had to increase well above its borrowing target.

KPMG (Klynveld Peat Marwick Goerdeler) the worldwide accounting and professional services firm, forecast that the UK GDP would decline by 2.6% for 2020, if the COVID-19 pandemic and the measures taken to contain it were successful by the summer of 2020. However a longer period of lockdown or a recurrence of infection with a second spike could lead to a 5.4% decline in GDP. The reduction in GDP is worse that the downturn in 2008 -2009 during the banking crisis of the time. Of course these projections are also dependent on satisfactory measures being enacted around the world to contain the pandemic. If the pandemic is contained and conditions remain favourable nationally and worldwide, it is possible that the GDP could grow by 1.7% in 2021.

Take car manufacturing. In May 2020 there was a 99% reduction in car production with only 197 cars having been produced. This is equivalent to a loss of £12 billion in revenue. The hospitality industry may never recover to pre-Covid-19 levels; it is predicted that 30,000 restaurants and pubs may shut up shop for good.

It is possible that the UK could experience an economic crash not seen since the Great Depression of the 1930's. Lockdown has led to reduction in general transport by greater than 60% and rail and Underground train use down by 95%. The use of roads by traffic has slumped to levels last seen in the 1950's. Add to this the empty airport terminals and fewer aeroplanes in the air and one gets a glimpse of the suspended animation that has affected the economy. And these activities are not likely to return to pre-lockdown levels anytime soon. This gives an idea of the massive reduction in economic activity. For example in a single 48-hour period in early July 2020 in the UK there was a loss of 11,000 jobs. This included jobs in Airbus Industries (aircraft manufacture), Upper Crust (catering), T M Lewin (clothing) etc. Large and small companies alike shed jobs as the end of the furlough period was approaching. The depression in economic activity is not confined to the UK alone. It amounts to the worst global depression in economic activity unrelated to global warfare.

The International Monetary Fund said that global GDP would fall by 3% in 2020 compared with a growth forecast of 3% before the onset of Covid-19. This is therefore the worst recession since the Great depression. A similar view is held by the Organisation of Economic Cooperation and Development (OECD). OECD is of the view that world economic output would fall by 6% this year, but that this would increase to 7.6% if a second spike in the infection occurs.

Different countries would be affected differently. India and China are likely to be affected to a lesser degree than other countries. However, the world over, OECD thinks that there would be long-lasting scars with a diminution of living standards, high unemployment and much reduced investment. In Europe France, Italy and Spain will be particularly badly affected.

What is the relevance of all of this information to the UK? As we have seen regards healthcare, a depressed economy is likely to affect the provision of health care adversely. With the preceding years of austerity in the NHS, it is difficult to see how a restart in safe healthcare could continue without a massive injection of cash that is targeted to areas of particular need like cancer care and cardiovascular disease.

Hard times lay ahead. The provision of safe and effective health and social care services, education, infrastructure projects etc is intricately linked with the performance of the economy. It is easy for anyone to say that government should spend more on health and social care without considering where money for any spend would come from. Money can only come from a well performing economy and from taxation. Governments cannot print money. But they can borrow for investment in healthcare. However, before going down this road, as with any borrowing, one needs to consider how borrowed money is likely to be paid back. Payback time will come. One would not like to be in a situation where the borrowing of today is left for settlement by future generations.

Race hate events and crimes have increased following the pandemic and lockdown. Phrases like 'China virus' or' Wuhan virus' do nothing to reduce the stigmatisation of sections of the population. The Monitoring Group (TMG) of the Institute of Race Relations has witnessed a large rise in racial abuse, harassment and violence against people of Chinese origin. These attacks are not confined to London but are being reported from cities across the UK. TMG has dedicated telephone lines with personnel working from home to help deal with racial attacks. It had reported a 160% increase in people contacting the TMG. It is feared that racial abuse would continue during lockdown and even afterwards.

Racial abuse may take many forms. Not only are there personal verbal and physical assaults on Chinese looking people and those of Asian descent who look like Chinese, but also property is vandalised, graffiti drawn on shop windows and on Chinese restaurants and takeaways. Chinese students at universities and in university hostels have also reported racial abuse. Not all attacks are on people of Chinese origin. Looking like a Chinese is sufficient for racial abuse to occur. There was a case in Orpington in Kent where a Japanese person was urinated upon. A member of the public spat at a student from Singapore in the London Underground. In another incident a man from Singapore was pushed and punched in Oxford Street in London. These persons just looked Chinese! These are deplorable and unforgivable act of depravity and inhumanity. Such acts shame all of us. We must always remind ourselves that we are better than this.

A regrettable aspect of racial abuse in these times is the abuse of key workers. Care workers, nurses, security guards, police etc are abused and attacked. These are people who are going about their usual business serving the community and are often serving the most vulnerable in society.

The failure of Police to act in these cases is lamentable. We saw the impotence of the Police during the 'Black Lives Matter' rallies. To allow the rioters in the rallies to damage property and not intervene is unpardonable. While bringing the perpetrators of violence to justice is the correct option, the failure to prevent violence in the first instance is inexcusable. In this respect the judiciary should also accept its due share of responsibility. Time and again its lenient sentencing policy has seen criminals get away with a literal 'slap on the wrist'. It sometimes appears that the UK is an ungovernable country because of the fear and failure of the Police to prosecute and the lax interpretation and enforcement of laws by the judiciary. There is no place for political correctness here. We had seen how earlier this year a Police Chief publicly apologised for looking aside when gangs of Asian men were abusing young girls. Political correctness stood in the way of justice and caused many young females to suffer unnecessarily.

Poverty in UK has been a recurrent social and political theme for many years. The Social Metrics Commission claims that there are, at present, 14.3 million people in poverty in the UK. This is made up of 8.3 million working-age adults, 4.6 million children and 1.3 million adults of pension age. The levels of poverty have remained much the same over the past 20 years and stands at 22% of the population. Of these people in poverty, 4 million are said to be in deep poverty. By deep poverty is meant that these people have an income that is at least 50% below the official breadline. For this group of people daily life is a struggle, with their meagre income hardly enough to meet the most basic of needs. Austerity and benefits cuts of recent years have severely affected the income of people in poverty. Reduction of almost £40 billion from benefits, tax credits etc have had a devastating impact, even before Covid-19 erupted on the scene.

It is estimated than ten million households in Britain have no savings, while another three million have less than £1,500 saved. Loss of work and therefore loss of any income during lockdown would push many people and households into deep poverty, where daily survival is a struggle.

Over 300,000 persons are homeless in the UK. Between four and five million people sleep rough on the streets each night in UK. This figure is double that which it was in 2010. The waste company Biffa, the Open University and the Chartered Institution of Wastes Management produced a report showing that many people sleep in waste disposal bins. This has led to an increase in the number of deaths and near misses when bins are being emptied. Seven people sleeping in bins are known to have been killed in the past five years and Biffa states that there have been 109 'near misses' between April and December 2019 involving people sleeping in or near bins. In the last 12 months 35% of waste companies reported finding people sleeping in bins compared to 21% in 2014. It is also noted that sleeping in bins is not only a winter problem but is found to occur all year round.

All people who are in poverty, those who lack of housing, rough sleepers etc are at great risk during lockdown. The lack of food, even periods of hunger, poor health and sanitation would make them vulnerable to Covid-19. If to this burden is added depression and other mental health issues one realises the enormous human cost, which may not all be related to the pandemic. But lockdown has added an obstacle, often insuperable, in the path of survival for many of these unfortunate members of society.

Across the world the effects of the pandemic is nothing short of disastrous. Disruption of routine services, often meagre in some places, would have an exponential adverse effect. In some parts of the Balkans for e.g. women have resorted to do-it-yourself abortions. One patient described how she used a glass full of red wine, boiled it, and dissolved in it a packet of aspirin, containing several tablets. She mixed it well until all the tablets were dissolved and drank the concoction. She hoped to induce a miscarriage. Disruption of services for patients with HIV/AIDS, tuberculosis etc would add to suffering and to the death toll. Polio is expected to return to some countries due to interruption of vaccination services. The United Nations' World Food Programme (WFP) said that the world is at a dangerous phase and is on the edge of a famine of 'biblical' proportions. It believes that 130 million additional people are at risk of starvation. This would be in addition to 130 million people who are already on the brink of starvation. Indirectly due to the pandemic, over a million children and 56,700 mothers could die.

Increased alcohol consumption during lockdown is a risk. Long periods of inactivity, boredom domestic and financial stress contribute to increased consumption. Also a myth has gained credence that alcohol protects against Covid-19. A common myth is that high strength alcohol is lethal to the coronavirus. This has led to people consuming greater quantities and higher strength of alcoholic drinks. The WHO responded to this by producing a public information leaflet stating that there is no validity in any such claim of protection from alcohol. The WHO information sheet draws the attention of people to the physical and psychological ill effects from alcohol. Alcohol also reduces the effect of the body's immune system, making it more susceptible to the virus. It is known from previous periods of mass stress that people who had drinking problems tended to drink more and this practice continued even for a year after the crisis had settled.

The frictions in and damage to international relationships is portrayed in the news regularly. Despite statements to the contrary, China is being held responsible for the worldwide spread of the infection and the havoc that it has unleashed. This has caused a strain in relationships with China. Claims and counter claims of responsibility have contributed to a low ebb in diplomatic relations. However many countries have strived to distance themselves from some of the more strident remarks that have surfaced during this time.

The European Union (EU) came under not inconsiderable strain during the pandemic. The EU was already in a difficult position prior to Covid-19. Its inability to have a coherent strategy for managing the migrant crisis led to some countries closing their borders. Similarly the EU's inability to arrive at any meaningful financial strategy to deal with the pandemic showed that the concept of union meant different things to different member countries. This could not have been more clearly seen than when Italy appeared isolated and left to its own devices in managing the pandemic.

o0:0o

'THE GOOD, THE BAD, THE UGLY'

Il buona, Il brutto, Il cattivo' - The Good, The Bad and The Ugly, was a sphagetti western film of the 1960's starring, Clint Eastwood, Le Van Cliff and Eli Wallach. These were three persons with varying knowledge of the subject, but who were united in their desire to find a buried treasure. The aim was clear. The characters of the three people played out on the screen as they pursued their own objectives.

As Covid-19 evolved and spread in the UK we have similarly seen on TV or read in newspapers how people across the whole social spectrum conducted themselves. The main objectives of personally avoiding infection and of reducing infection in the community were not lost sight of. But in the process, people had their own wishes that they displayed. Most of what people did was good and altruistic. Some things that we saw and read about could be called bad as they inflicted pain and suffering on others. Several things we heard about were ugly because they tended to show personal gain or vanity while the majority of people were enduring a difficult time.

The opening of the Nightingale Hospital in London on 3rd April 2020 by video link was a source of reassurance to the public. This 4000 bed hospital was erected in a few months, complete with all the facilities including piped oxygen. However we later learned that it had to reject admission to several patients due to staffing shortages. This was likely to be a problem given the size of the hospital and what it was supposed to provide. There was no possibility of all 4000 beds in the London

Nightingale Hospital being occupied at the same time by gravely ill patients who all needed ventilator support. This would have required a vast army of medical professionals of all necessary skills with all the necessary equipment including several thousand ventilators.

One needs to look at the concept of the Nightingale Hospitals. At the time they were planned, the UK faced the prospect of there being a surge in cases of Covid-19. The UK was behind Italy by a few weeks in the peak of the illness. And we were aware of the strain being placed on health services in Italy by the rapid increase in cases of Covid-19 and the numbers of severely ill patients who needed to be in hospital. Many of these patients needed ventilation. Also the Nightingale Hospitals were envisaged as over-spill facilities which could relieve pressure on intensive care units in other hospitals in and around London and elsewhere. Due to better local planning, it turned out that most of the hospitals in London were able to increase their intensive care capacity and so were able to deal with increases in demand. However, Northwick Park Hospital in north-west London was not able to cope with the patient load due to coronavirus. It intended transferring about 30 patients to the Nightingale Hospital in London. But staffing issues in the latter meant that the transfers did not go through. Northwick Park Hospital had to close its doors to admissions due to pressure on beds, intensive care facilities and on staff. Some other hospitals like the Royal Free Hospital, the Royal London Hospital and North Middlesex Hospital were not able to transfer some of their patients to the Nightingale Hospital. Weston General Hospital in Weston-super-Mare, Somerset, also closed due to staff being positive to the virus. However neighbouring hospitals were able to step in and compensate such that the need for the Nightingale Hospitals diminished.

While some may criticise the creation of Nightingale Hospitals as a waste of resources, we need to look at the concept of these hospitals in the light of the threat from a rapidly spreading pandemic. We were witness to the threat to health services in Italy. As was said, the NHS needed 'to plan for the worst and hope for the best'. As it turned out London hospitals were largely able to cope with the increased work generated by Covid-19. We also know that the government was trying to increase the availability of ventilators to help manage a worst case scenario, if it happened. This was good planning.

Apart from the fact that the NHS was not overwhelmed by Covid-19 there were other reasons why the hospitals were not used. Patients who were very ill form Covid-19 often were at risk of or also had failure of other organs in the body like to kidneys. At the outset, Covid-19 was seen as mainly a respiratory infection and that the essential need would be for respiratory support. That is the need for ventilation until the patient's lungs could recover sufficiently to breath unaided. But with time the nature of Covid-19 infection became clearer and the medical profession learned and continues to learn more about the disease with each passing day. Especially we learned that it is a disease that affected multiple systems in the body, also called a multi-system disorder. For e.g. many patients have a great risk of thrombosis or clots in the legs, lungs and elsewhere. Kidney failure, if it occurs, would have also needed treatment and support. The Nightingale Hospitals as originally envisaged were for managing patients whose main need is for ventilation. These hospitals were not initially designed for supporting patients with multi-organ failure. However, if there was an overwhelming pandemic it is not impossible to imagine that the Nightingale Hospitals would have been re-purposed to also deal with some patients who needed other means of treatment apart from ventilation.

Looking at the totality of the evolving nature of Covid-19 it was always prudent to conceive of the Nightingale Hospitals.

However there are always lessons to be learned from plans for events of this nature. Not only buildings but also relevant, skilled personnel and equipment need to be factored in during pandemic planning. Surge planning is a complex logistical exercise where all aspects from prevention to treatment and even the dignified disposal of those who die need to be considered so that a comprehensive 'system of systems' could be in place at short notice.

The need for ventilators was evident early on during the outbreak of the infection. This need became an emergency in itself when we saw what was happening in Italy. A shortage of ventilators was paramount in Italy's ability to deal with patients who needed support with their breathing. As the UK was a few weeks behind Italy in the peak of the virus, it was natural and vital for the government to seek help in obtaining ventilators in time for any surge in cases. British manufacturers responded to calls by the Prime Minister and the Government to help in producing ventilators. Vauxhall,

Rolls-Royce, Jaguar, Airbus are some of the engineering companies that responded positively. Vauxhall which was due to shut down on 27th March was planning to use its paint shop to help in production of ventilators because of the availability of better controlled environment in these sites.

Blease is a company in the UK that has been making its Nippy ventilators for over 25 years. It increased its staff and moved to a seven day working week even though other companies were in lockdown mode.

The Ventilator UK Challenge Consortium came into existence. It is led by Dick Elsy, CEO of High Value Manufacturing Catapult, which is a group of research centres in the UK that helps manufacturing companies.

On 17th April the Medicines and Healthcare products Regulatory Agency (MHRA) approved Penlon's Prima ES02 model ventilator for UK hospitals. And on 22nd April the first batch of Penlon ventilators arrived at Nightingale Hospitals in London and Bristol.

Dyson produced 10,000 ventilators but by the time they were available, the need for them had lessened. But the company hoped that other countries may find a use for their ventilators.

Gtech based in Worcester was another manufacturing company that rose to the challenge of producing ventilators. Gtech was informed by the government on 20th March to proceed with manufacture. However, on 26th March the company was advised by the government's coordinating group not to proceed with manufacture of the ventilators, again apparently due to diminished need for them. The company yet planned to complete the design of the machine and publish it so that other countries may benefit. The Chief Executive, Nick Grey, praised his staff for their response to the needs of the time.

In late March 2020 engineers form University College London teamed up with Mercedes, the car manufacturer, to produce a variant of the CPAP machine that can be used in Covid-19 patients. Continuous Positive Airways Pressure (CPAP) delivers oxygen or air into the lungs under pressure without the need for a tube inserted into the windpipe. Ventilation does the same, but oxygen is delivered into the lungs through a tube (endotracheal tube) inserted into the windpipe (trachea). CPAP does not need a tube in the windpipe. It had been used in Italy and in China in Covid-19 patients. The MHRA has recommended its use on patients.

Many companies also responded to the shortage of personal protective equipment (PPE) like masks, goggles, wipers, gowns, surgical scrubs etc. PPE is vital in medical and social care to prevent transmission of germs form one person to another. This is very important for healthcare and other frontline works. If these personnel fell ill, the numbers of them who would be available to care for patients would be reduced. This could have serious consequences for the care of patients and those in care homes.

Many companies across the world responded by producing PPE and hand sanitiser solution. LVMH, L'Oreal, Zara, Guerlain, Prada are some big names who have diverted some of their productions lines to serve the needs of the time.

By 16th April BAE engineering had delivered to the NHS 24,000 units of their 3-D printed new face shields with another 40,000 due for delivery the following week. Amtico, the Coventry based flooring manufacturer, used its production facilities to make up to 20,000 protective face shields a day. They are using their specialist skills to ensure the 'best balance between flexibility and rigidity' when their face shields are used by NHS frontline staff.

Barbour, the clothing and accessories company based in South Shields has supplied the NHS with gowns and other PPE. Burberry used it's trench coat factory in Castleford, in the north of England, to make protective gowns for healthcare workers. Burberry also declined to use the government's furlough scheme for its employees. And to its credit Burberry directors took a 20% pay reduction from April to June 2020 and the money was used for charity. The group also said its senior leaders and directors will take a voluntary 20% pay cut from April through June, with the directors' 20% donated to a charity fund.

David Nieper, ladies fashion wear producers, had to furlough their staff. But sewing staff returned to their Alfreton factories to help make scrubs etc for the NHS. They initially offered their services to the NHS but these efforts were frustrated by slow NHS bureaucracy and red tape. They gave up on the central bureaucracy and dealt directly with two University Hospital Trusts in Leicestershire and Derbyshire. In total they produced 5000 scrubs for nine hospitals in the two Trusts. With two sewing factories and two shifts patterns, the company was able to work safely while observing social distancing rules in the factories. Work started over the Easter weekend and at the time of writing the firm had produced

30,000 pieces of PPE. This was made up of 16,000 clinical hoods, 7000 scrubs and 19,000 reusable gowns. The reusable gowns can be washed, sterilised and used over and over again cleanly and safely for over 50 times. The company also said that on Thursdays, 'clap day', the sewing teams, whether working in the factory or in their own homes, wore blue in honour of the heroes of healthcare that served the nation during the Covid-19 crisis.

The Caring Foundation is named after the tycoon Richard Caring. Richard Caring owns several clubs and restaurants spread around the UK and Ireland. While these businesses were in lockdown, he used the available facilities to provide meals to children, vulnerable communities and unemployed people across the UK and Ireland. More than a thousand staff worked in kitchens and provided food in Birmingham, Belfast, Cardiff, Dublin, Brighton and London. Richard Caring compares the current situation with Covid-19 to the Blitz during World War II, but magnified ten times. He makes a plea for decisive action by the government if the country is to avoid having to face the possibility of an unemployment rate as high as 25%.

Many individuals and local organisations responded to help with PPE. The Daily Mail campaign showed what can be achieved when one taps into the basic humanitarian spirit of the British public. Time and time again one has seen the enormous responses to appeals by the UK's Disasters Emergency Committee. The desire to help runs deep in the human heart and we have witnessed that during the Covid-19 crisis.

These are some of the examples of how large and medium sized firms have responded to the needs of the NHS. But small producers and private individuals too have risen to the challenge. Maidstone Sewing Group for the NHS is one example. Caroline Barton started sewing bags so that staff like her mother, who is a nurse, could place their uniforms at the end of a shift. She then formed a sewing group which at the beginning of May had produced items for Maidstone and Tunbridge Wells hospitals. The 20,000 items produced consisted of 9,000 bags, 5,000 headbands, 4,000 scrub caps, 1,300 scrubs and gowns.

Many companies returned or are planning to return money to the government, which they received under the employee furlough scheme. This is money that was paid out by the government to help support companies and to avoid large-scale redundancies. There was neither an obligation on the part of companies to return the money nor was there a linked claw-back scheme where the money would have eventually been claimed from a company. The Telegraph and Spectator newspapers which are both owned by the Barclay brothers plan to return money that they had received. Bunzl, a FTSE 100 company makes and sells packaging to supermarkets and supplies hospitals with gloves and gowns. It plans to return the money it received under the scheme. So also the fantasy gaming company, Games Workshop plans to return money to the government. The company is behind the 'War hammer' toy soldiers. Ikea has said it would return money in all nine countries that it received support from, following better than expected company results. Bellway the house builder did not take money from the government under the scheme. Some other companies too have not participated in the scheme, having declined to accept government aid in this respect.

Talking about returning money to the government, Andrew Neill of the Spectator said 'we do this not to set an example for other companies to follow, but because we can afford to do so'. Facing a financial disaster during lockdown, resulting from reduction in sales and loss of advertising revenue, the newspaper initially decided to seek financial help from the government. But it was able to increase its number of subscribers and was in a position to return a profit for the year. Some have expressed doubts about the altruism of companies which chose to return money to the Exchequer. Non-receipt of money from the government or returning what was received allows a company to manage its accounts the way it chooses to do. A company could therefore pay dividends, pay bonuses to staff etc without being the subject of too much scrutiny. Those businesses that accepted taxpayers' money are likely to face much greater scrutiny in this respect, if they are seen to be rewarding shareholders or paying out hefty bonuses to any staff. So this should be! However, the Chief Executive of the construction company Taylor Wimpey, said that 'it feels right' to return money that it had received stating that the company had a strong balance sheet.

But while this was happening there were about 850 employees who reported their respective employers to the Her Majesty's Revenue and Customs (HMRC) for fraud over the furlough scheme. Under the scheme the government paid 80% of an employee's wages up to a maximum of £2500 per month. However to be eligible, the employee must not be working for the employer. But several employees have informed HMRC that their employer wanted them to work while being in receipt of money under the Coronavirus Job Retention Scheme.

Admiral was the first motor vehicle insurer in the UK to refund customers part of the premiums paid because of limited or no driving during lockdown. Admiral planned to return £110m to its policyholders– a £25 refund for each car and van it insured. Other vehicle insurers followed suit.

When we are ill and admitted to hospital we hope that our family and friends would be there to visit us, talk to us, cheer us up in our dark periods and generally help us back to better health. They would be there to accompany us back home where would be welcomed. Unfortunately this is not possible with Covid-19. A person with Covid-19 who is admitted to hospital is consigned to spend those days alone. Surrounded they are, round the clock with caring persons whose faces they cannot see. This is the nature of the illness and the risk of infection with Covid-19. The patient with Covid-19 becomes, in many respects, an 'untouchable'.

The word 'untouchable' has many connotations. It may mean that such a person is above the law or is so good at what he or she does, like a sportsman. The 'untouchable' in American law enforcement referred to officers who were as fearless as they were not susceptible to bribery.

Untouchable in the old Indian cast system referred to those persons of a lower social class, although this has largely disappeared from Indian society.

Covid-19 has brought a new meaning to the word 'untouchable'. Patients with Covid-19 are at risk of infecting others. They are 'untouchable' in a most benign sense of the word, implying that they are a risk to others.

So patients with Covid-19 are alone in their world of thoughts and fears. They are not allowed family, friends or visitors. A covid-19 ward in a hospital is an isolation ward.

Patients who unfortunately die of Covid-19, do so alone and afraid with none of their loved ones to see them or comfort them in their last days. The immense sadness of this kind of parting for the patient and family is indescribable.

The fundamental human need to be close to loved ones is denied in Covid-19. The patient is cut off from his world of family and loved ones, at a time when he needs them most.

Into this terrible emotional void came Dr.Louise Rose from Kings College Hospital, London and Dr. Joel Meyer from Guys and St. Thomas' Hospital, also in London. They developed a communication app that facilitates virtual visits by loved ones to a patient in hospital. It is called LifeLines. The two doctors worked closely together and speedily to develop the app because of the harrowing scenes of patients being left alone and dying alone. They take a computer tablet to the patient who can then talk with family and / or the family can see the patient, if he is on a ventilator. Staff can use the app to keep the family informed of progress. Importantly, staff can discuss prognosis with the family, especially if the patient is deteriorating and not likely to survive. Although this is not an ideal means of communicating when death is near. Communication at this time of life is best done face-to-face; this is not possible with Covid-19. The app serves as a useful intermediary at a vulnerable time for patient and family.

The role of volunteers in the life of the country is a continuing story of service to people, communities and the nation at large. So it is no wonder that there was an incredible response when the Health Secretary, Matt Hancock, appealed in March 2020 for 250,000 volunteers to help during the crisis. Their primary purpose would be to support the approximately 1.5 million people who were advised to 'shield' themselves at home when lockdown came in. Those who had to 'shield' invariably have underlying conditions like lung disease, cancer, bone marrow cancers, diabetes etc, which make them at greater risk of Covid -19 and at a greater risk of dying from it. They were advised to stay at home and not to leave home. Shielding was partially lifted on the 1st June 2020. This meant that these persons were invariably in total 'house arrest' for their own safety. The role of volunteers was to support those who are at home – helping with shopping, dealing with their health care needs and especially talking to them. Some of these persons may be living alone with hardly any contact with others, even in normal times.

There is another group of volunteers that one seldom hears about. These are the healthy persons who volunteer to participate in drug and vaccine trials related to Civid-19. A study by the University of Oxford and the Wellcome Trust in association with colleagues in Bangkok, Thailand was investigating the use of the anti-malarial drug, hydrocychloroquine, in Covid-19. Subsequently there were the vaccine trials and especially the 'Challenger' trials. In a Challenge study a person is given a Covid-19 vaccine which is hoped would provide immunity. A few weeks later the person is then infected with live coronavirus. This tests the ability of the body to overcome the virus and protect the person, if the previously administered vaccine had worked. Persons taking part in such a trail would be under close medical supervision and be in quarantine. Challenger trials have been used in the past for vaccines against influenza (flu), typhoid etc. It is not a new concept. But it requires brave and altruistic volunteers.

The first week in June of each year is traditionally Volunteers Week. This is a period when the country recognises its volunteers, thanks them for their selflessness and celebrates the presence of volunteers in our midst. This year, in 2020, the Duchess of Cornwall, who is the President of the Voluntary Service, acknowledged the immense contribution of volunteers in saying "This year in particular, we owe a great debt of thanks to all our wonderful volunteers, who have stepped forward in astonishing numbers, pulling together to support those affected by COVID-19'. She referred to volunteers as the 'backbone' of the country, echoing the words of Sir Wilfred Trotter more than one hundred years before. At end of Volunteer Week, on 6th June 2020, Her Majesty, The Queen shared words of thanks to 'all those who give themselves so freely and selflessly in the service of others'. Her Majesty wrote 'It is inspiring to reflect on the many thousands of people, who through their acts of generosity and kindness have achieved so much for the greater good'.

Thursday 23rd April was an important day in the Covid-19 journey. On this day the first human trials of a vaccine against Covid-19 commenced in Oxford. Five hundred people volunteered for the trail. Of this number 250 people were given the vaccine and 250 were comparators who did not get the vaccine. Instead, the comparators were given a meningitis vaccine which has no effect on Covid-19. This is a double blind trial where none of the volunteers knew what they were being injected with – either the Covid-19 vaccine or the meningitis vaccine. They were therefore 'blind' to what they received. Also the researchers doing the trial did not know which volunteers got the vaccine and which did not. So the researchers were also 'blind'; hence a double blind trial. This prevents bias in interpretation of the eventual results and would help proper statistical analysis of the efficacy or not of the vaccine.

In Belfast, Northern Ireland, it was reported on 6th May 2020 that the health service there was able to do 30 kidney transplants during a two week period of the pandemic. Most non-urgent NHS work had ceased across the United Kingdom during the lockdown. This included cessation of most routine surgery including transplant surgery. But in Belfast hospitals the kidney transplant units remained open. This allowed surgical teams to carry out a record-breaking five kidney transplants in a single 24-hour period and continued this rate of transplants on several days. It was a remarkable and 'unbelievable' achievement according to Dr. Aisling Courtney, a kidney transplant consultant. The transplant teams remain deeply grateful to the deceased donors of kidneys. The availability of kidneys allowed the transplants operations to proceed. The operations were 'very tiring work but, but we just keep operating and operating," according to transplant surgeon Tim Brown. This achievement is astounding at the height of the pandemic!

Now here is particularly good news. Not surprisingly lockdown has contributed to a reduction in some crimes. Market Harborough is a town in the county of Leicestershire in England. It has a population of about 90,000 people. Market Harborough had seen the biggest fall in crime. The number of reported crimes fell from 443 in March 2019 to 49 in Mach 2020. Of all crimes, personal theft showed the biggest fall. This fell to less than a third of its usual number. Shoplifting was down by 54% but this again, is not unexpected in the climate of lockdown with virtually all shops being closed. Reporting of rape was also less but antisocial behaviour showed a rise during lockdown. According to Police, during a four week period in lockdown there were 178,000 incidents of anti-social behaviour in England and Wales. This is a rise of 59% compared to the same period in 2019. Car crimes in general were lower in lockdown. The Home Secretary said that overall the numbers of crimes has diminished during lockdown. Police reported receiving fewer calls to 999 and 101. The numbers of cases brought to the attention of Police relating to missing persons and mental health issues have also dropped. These two areas are often difficult to interpret from simple statistics alone. We are likely to learn more about mental health issues during lockdown.

The effect of the global lockdown on the environment is nothing short of dramatic. It is estimated that emissions of carbon dioxide gas dropped by 17% compared to figures for the same period in 2019. The low levels reached in lockdown were last seen in 2006. The 17% reduction in emissions is equivalent to 17 million tonnes of carbon dioxide. In China alone there was a 25% reduction in carbon emissions in February 2020. The reduction in atmospheric pollution and improvement in air quality was significant enough to allow people in North India to see the Himalayas for the first time in their lives; for the first time the mountain range had been visible in the last 30 years. The Taj Mahal could be seen in its pristine glory without the smog that often clouded over it; it was reported that swans had returned to Venetian canals. Of course this impressive reduction in pollution is solely due to lockdown and as such is not likely to be permanent. But if the majority of us could use for e.g. alternative means of transport, it may be possible nationally and globally to reduce toxic emissions.

In the UK the amount of tiny particles that pollute the air reduced by 30%-50% in London, Birmingham, Bristol and Cardiff. In Manchester, York and Belfast levels of tiny particles reduced by 25%. These findings show that reduction in travel help to reduce air pollution and to improve the quality of the air that we breathe.

The same reductions were seen in the amount of nitric oxide in the air.

The reductions in motor vehicle use and the drastic reduction in aeroplane travel have contributed to global improvements in air quality.

The improvement in air quality is not only aesthetically and visually pleasing. It has had an impact on health and mortality. The British Lung Foundation says that people with asthma have had fewer symptoms during lockdown, with one in six people having noticed improvements in their health. Children's health has fared even better with one in five parents saying that their children's asthma or other lung condition was better during lockdown.

The British Lung Foundation says that these findings show how important it is for us to look after our lungs.

These findings should prompt governments around the world to work to reduce air pollution. Air pollution contributes to 40,000 deaths per year in the UK.

The Centre for International Climate Research in Oslo claims that improvements in air quality as a result of lockdown could lead to a reduction in premature deaths of between 50,000 to 100,000. Research from Stanford University, California say that improvements in air quality in China may have saved 4000 children below the age of 5 years and 74,000 people above the age of 70 years.

Lockdown may just have shown us how quickly the natural world around us can adapt, recover, repair and thrive when we limit our encroachment into their environments.

Covid-19 has conspired with nature to provide a brief glimpse of our beautiful plant, Earth, our home. Covid-19 has caused much suffering and death. Many of those who died from Covid-19, did so because their lungs became so congested with fluid due to inflammation. The lungs were choked and there was very little spare good lung to help breathing. These patients needed ventilation until their lungs improved and became 'unchoked' as it were. A ventilator is a kind of artificial lung which forces air into the lungs. Stop for a moment and hold that thought – 'choking lungs'. That is what we have been doing to our planet. We are progressively and slowly but surely choking it and the end is inevitable. When the Amazon forest was being cleared, politicians and people from around the world protested that the 'lungs of the world' were being destroyed or 'choked'. As Covid-19 sadly choked some people to death, future generations will hold us responsible for choking the planet. After seeing what our world could be but still continuing to choke it, we would stand accused of unpardonable folly. We were given a beautiful home, shown how we could make it better and we still chose to destroy it.

The human Cognitive Revolution took place 70,000 years ago. When that happened, homo changed to home sapiens. The development of intelligence and communication allowed man to encroach, in leaps and bounds, on the flora and fauna of the world. It also led eventually to the Industrial Revolution, which was the ultimate driver for the pollution that we see today. Covid-19 has shown what a 'un-polluted' or a 'less-polluted' world may look like. We can now grasp the nettle or forever the planet would be increasingly polluted.

There were and continue to be many more stories of human kindness during lockdown. Not all could be included in this brief description. But one stands out for the drive of one person coupled with the magnanimity and generosity of many others. It is of course the story of Captain Tom Moore. Thomas Moore is 99 years old. With a view to his 100th birthday on 30th April 2020, he conceived of the idea on 6th April 2020 of raising £1000 for NHS charities. He began walking in his back garden with the aid of his walking frame. He did this wearing his army uniform and adorned with his military medals. He reached his target of £1000 on 10th April and as his birthday was still some days away raised his target, first to £5000 and then to £500,000. People from around the world became aware of what he was doing and contributed to his collection. On the day of his birthday he had collected in excess of £32 million and his JustGiving page was closed.

Michael Ball sang 'You'll Never Walk Alone' for Capt Tom on BBC breakfast TV. Capt. Tom's duet with Michael Ball was made into a record and all proceeds from the sale of the record would also go to NHS Charities Together. The record reached the Number 1 spot on the Singles Chart on 24th April. Tom Moore became the oldest person to reach the top singles spot. He was made Honorary Colonel and was awarded the Pride of Britain award. 'Colonel' Tom Moore was knighted and became Sir Thomas Moore on 20th May 2020.

NHS Charities Together distributes money to charities for use at local levels. Some of the money has been used to provide rest spaces, sleep pods and well-being packs for staff. Money has been used to purchase computer tablets so that patients can contact family and friends. Money would also be used to provide mental support to families and staff.

Capt. Tom's achievement is spectacular compared to those who have sought to take out than give to the country and the NHS. The words of John Fitzgerald Kennedy are not lost here – ' ask not what your country can do for you, but what you can do for your country'. Perhaps all of us should ask ourselves the same question, especially big business and those with means, who have chosen to take rather than to give!

The story of Capt. Tom Moore is the stuff of legends!

Prior to the lockdown when life was going on as normal many people had planned and booked airline travel and holidays. Suddenly these were not to be. What happens to the monies that travellers had already paid to holiday companies? It is obvious that in the unusual circumstances of the lockdown a full refund would be made.

There is a legal obligation of travel companies to refund monies to their customers. But this was not easy and the companies were not as forthcoming as it would seem. Some companies refused to provide refunds while others set out providing vouchers or credit notes to customers. The latter are against the law which requires a refund to be made, when requested. Besides, the alternatives may not be acceptable to customers who may not wish to travel at some future date. There is also the possibility that credit notes and vouchers may not be worth the paper they are written on if the respective companies go out of business.

There is no obligation on the part of the traveller to accept anything other than a refund of money paid. Under EU law customers must be refunded within 14 days if the holiday is cancelled. There is no doubt that the travel industry is under enormous financial pressure due to lockdown. But as Which magazine's Rory Boland wrote it cannot be the responsibility of customers to help prop up airlines and travel firms. Customers too are under considerable financial pressure with lower or no income during the lockdown.

In the initial weeks of lockdown it was estimated that £7 billion had been paid by UK customers to airlines.

It was particularly unfortunate when in the middle of April 2020, Novak Djokovic, the reigning Wimbledon champion expressed his opposition to vaccination. In a Facebook conversation he said 'personally I am opposed to vaccination and I wouldn't want to be forced by someone to take a vaccine in order to be able to travel,'; 'But if it becomes compulsory, what will happen? I will have to make a decision'. This was a time when scientists and researchers around the world were working to develop an effective vaccine against the coronavirus to protect the public.

At about the same time in April 2020 the WHO was discussing issues about vaccine and the eventual availability of it to all irrespective of national wealth etc.

Even prior to Covid-19 the world was facing a resurgence of infectious disease like measles, which could be prevented by a safe and effective vaccine. The anti-vaccination lobby has been successful in persuading parents of the merit of its case and of the dangers of vaccination. Many parents have bought into this narrative and prevented their children from being vaccinated. Much as one would disagree with the views of those who are against vaccination, one would defend to the hilt their right to express those views. However parents and carers and other adults may not get a balanced view of the overwhelming merits of vaccination and so they may be denied the ability to make an informed choice on the matter.

Mr. Djokovic is probably a role model for many in the world. Young impressionable persons are likely to be influenced by his views. It is regrettable that he chose this particular time to express his views on vaccination. It is not as if vaccination is immediately available against Covid-19 or that it was required for international travel or that competitive tennis was likely to commence in the near future.

The combination of home working, poorly protected office sites, fast tracking of payments without appropriate checks etc provides ample opportunities for fraudsters. Procurement of supplies for the health service was likely to be fast-tracked because of the need to obtain material urgently. The usual checks and balances may be bypassed in the apparent interest of patient safety. The National Crime Agency in the UK has alerted individuals and organisation to the risks of fraud and scams. The Security Minister, James Brokenshire, warned the public that criminals are callous and would use the public's vulnerability at this time to enrich themselves. There had been examples of online shopping scams where people had paid for face masks, gloves, hand sanitiser etc., which never arrived. There had also been examples of criminals selling false Cocid-19 testing kits. These had not been medically approved and therefore results obtained from these test were unlikely to be valid. Even reputable professionals may have been selling approved test kits but at enormously inflated prices.

Computer fraud was also likely to increase and the public has been warned not to share sensitive details like passwords with anyone. This is basic safety advice, but in the current climate and with fear being an ingredient of daily life, there was a likelihood of people falling prey to a scam. We were advised to be wary of unsolicited mail and special offers. If an offer looked too good to be true, it was almost certainly unlikely to be true! It is a scam.

By early April 2020 there were over 500 scams connected with

Covid-19. The common ingredient in most of these cases had been fear of the pandemic and the accompanying uncertainty about the future.

A common scam starts with unsolicited calls or emails seeking help with money being sought for a fighting fund for Covid-19. Or, money to purchase life-saving equipment for the NHS. News on TV, in newspapers and public discussion heightened anxiety in public about how the NHS was coping. These concerns about shortages of PPE for e.g. are being used by fraudsters to highlight the desperate plight of the NHS and to plead for help. The elderly who were shielding at home because of their perceived vulnerability to Covid-19 were simultaneously vulnerable to scams related to Covid-19. Impersonation as a volunteer who is willing and ready to help someone who is shielding is not uncommon. Theft of personal possessions and fraud has resulted.

Among the many scams during Covid-19 and lockdown, perhaps the worst is those persons trying to make money from attempting to supply vital medical equipment to the NHS. New businesses sprung up masquerading as healthcare suppliers. These businesses were selling equipment like PPE to hospital and care homes at hugely inflated prices. About the same time a man from Wirral in northwest England was jailed for 28 months in June for theft of PPE. He stole the material from the company he was working for and sole them on eBay. The material he stole was valued at £30,000. While passing sentence the judge commented that the NHS was 'crying out' for the equipment at the time.

In April 2020 alone there were over 9000 'sextortion' phishing scams. In this type of scam the victim's password is known to the scammer who, not uncommonly, declares it to the victim. The demand is for payment in Bitcoin rather than standard currency. Sextortion first appeared in 2018. 'Sextortion' is a form of pornographic scam. The Journal of Interpersonal Violence defines it as sexual extortion where there is ' the threatened dissemination of explicit, intimate, or embarrassing images of a sexual nature without consent, usually for the purpose of procuring additional images, sexual acts, money, or something else'. The cybercriminal sends an email to a victim claiming to have records of pornography that the victim has been viewing. The criminal may also claim to know the victims passwords. This is usually false or they may have an old password or a telephone number. This information may have been available in and obtained from the dark internet. Harassment of the victim continues with payment being demanded. The cybercriminal often does not have any evidence to support what is being claimed. But the victim does not know this. The purpose of the email is to engender vulnerability and to intimidate the victim into paying. The University of Michigan states that sextortion is a risk to children and to adults. The University advises everyone not to send compromising images of themselves to another, whoever they may be and to turn off web cameras when not in use. It is also good practice not to open attachments from people one does not know.

The Pensions Regulatory and the Financial Conduct Authority had advised the public not to make decisions about pensions in the current climate of uncertainty in almost every walk of life. Rash decisions, they say, are not good decisions. Also, discussions with any new advisor are best avoided during this period. The Financial Conduct Authority (FCA) has warned the public to be wary, especially the elderly who are vulnerable to scams affecting their pensions and investments. The public are warned to be suspicious of unsolicited emails and telephone calls. We are also warned not to succumb to exaggerated claims of financial gain. These are unlikely to be true. Isolation during lockdown is a fertile ground for criminals.

As far as smuggling drugs is concerned there is no human crisis that would limit this activity. On the contrary every crisis provides an opportunity to exploit it for the perverse ends of drug smugglers. No human suffering would stand in the way of drug runners and smugglers. It was reported in April 2020 that 14kg of cocaine with a value of £1 million pounds was smuggled into the UK in a van driven by a Polish national. The haul of cocaine was contained in boxes of face masks which had been labelled as vital medical equipment. Nothing can describe the public revulsion at this, when, at the same time, the NHS was facing a shortage of PPE and people were dying from Covid-19.

Drug trafficking arrests in London went up by 55% between the middle of March 2020 and the middle of April 2020.County lines in the UK are drug distribution networks where criminal gangs use vulnerable people and even children to send drugs from the cities to rural areas. Contacts are established using special telephone lines. In 2018, the National Crime Agency identified 1500 drug trafficking routes in the county lines network with an annual turnover of £500 million. It involved about 25,000 people. Operation 'Orochi' by the Metropolitan Police involved identifying the main traffickers and producing them in courts for drug trafficking. Eighteen 'drug lords' were identified and their distribution lines shut down. The eighteen leaders were jailed as a result of this successful operation. The Police have been able to shut down 87 county lines. Of the 18 cases that have gone to the courts so far, all the defendants pleaded guilty and received a total of more than 50 years of imprisonment. One of those sent to prison for five years had only recently been released from prison after serving a nine year sentence for being the head of a county line. Another person who was jailed for five years was running his county line from a bedroom in London where police found heroin, cocaine, knives and a canister of CS gas.

As always in crises like the Covid-19 pandemic there is fear and confusion. These provide a fertile ground for those who are prepared to peddle conspiracy theories. Conspiracy thrives at times like this. And into this space migrated the likes of David Icke. David Icke claimed that there is nothing dangerous about Covid19. It is not the serious disease that it is claimed to be. He views lockdown as the imposition of a kind of martial law designed on false pretexts to curtail our freedoms. In his view lockdown is not about protecting the vulnerable but about infringing our basic human rights.

David Icke quoted information from the UK government website document 'Status of Covid-19' to justify his opinion that this was a mild, benign illness. The UK government maintained that 'as of March 19th 2020 Covid-19 is no longer considered to be a high consequence infectious disease (HCID) in the UK'. This was before the gravity of the illness was recognised and before the death toll started to increase, nationally and internationally.

On his website David Icke maintains that the Covid-19 pandemic is being used by the ruling elites to subjugate the population. He writes that Covid-19 is less of a threat that seasonal flu. According to him, countries are using fear of Covid-19 as a means of manipulating the public into subservience. This may be achieved by lockdown, fines, imprisonment and in some countries even by death.

He disseminated the view that the virus originated in the USA.

Both YouTube and Facebook took down messages from David Icke.

YouTube deleted his channel because it violated company's rules about the coronavirus. He had claimed that Covid-19 is a hoax. The Centre for Countering Digital Hate (CCDH) commended YouTube for its action.

Coughing and spitting has been used as a weapon by some people against police officers and care workers. One person was sent to prison for a year and another to six months in prison for spitting at a nurse. At one time there were 300 reported attacks on Police and emergency staff.

The Royal College of Nursing appealed to the public to be supportive of nurses after some nurses in the community had been spat at and called 'disease spreaders'.

Trevor Belle aged 61 was a taxi driver who was spat at by a passenger who owed him £9 in taxi fare. Following this event Mr. Belle felt unwell and was admitted to hospital. He was in hospital for three weeks and died of Covid-19, Mr. Belle had just become a grandfather.

At Mile End Underground station in London, a man without a ticket spat at a female passenger who intervened after he demanded that staff open the barriers.

One of the unfortunate but not entirely unexpected negative aspects of Covid-19 is the racial stereotyping of people that has followed the onset of the pandemic. This is a 'Chinese' disease, so some claimed or the 'Wuhan' virus. Many people associated Covid-19 with Asia – it is an 'Asian' disease. As a result of such unfounded compartmentalising of the disease, people of Chinese and Asian descent have been subjected to racism. People who even look Chinese but are not Chinese are also abused. Xenophobia has taken hold in many quarters.

There are about 400,000 people of Chinese origin living in Britain. Some have them have settled in the UK and have been living here for many years. They are distributed across the country in London, Manchester, Newcastle etc. Many cities have a Chinese quarter. The Chinese population is an integral part of cities and local communities. There are a large proportion of Chinese students in universities across the UK. The racial attacks against these people have varied from verbal abuse to physical violence.

Some examples of what have happened are shocking. A group of Chinese people were assaulted in Southampton. They were wearing face masks at the time of the assault. In another case a Chinese student's jaw was broken in an assault. In one incident a trainee lawyer was rendered unconscious after being knocked down by an attacker. She was only trying to defend a Chinese friend, who was with her at the time, from racial abuse.

A Chinese community group in Birmingham received a Facebook message that read - "The disgusting, barbaric animal cruelty you people do - you all deserve to get the virus."

The term 'maskophobia' arose following Covid-19. It is the fear of people wearing face masks. Face masks are worn regularly by large numbers of people in countries in Asia. It is often worn there because of the high levels of atmospheric pollution. But when Covid-19 emerged in the UK, people wearing masks were identified as Chinese and therefore carriers of the virus. Ignorance and intolerance led to racial attacks. Out of fear, many Chinese students chose to fly back to their homes in China. They had to pay exaggerated airline prices to secure whatever seats that was available on aeroplanes that were still flying. Chinese students expected more severe measures to be introduced in the UK to help combat the virus than the initial advice about hand washing etc. Fear of the virus and fear of attacks led many to flee the UK back to the safety of their homes in China.

A Chinese researcher in London stated that most of the attacks were associated with wearing of masks and from fear of people wearing masks.

There are about 125,000 Chinese students in the UK. One spoke for most Chinese students in saying that they chose to come to the UK because of its values of tolerance, equality and diversity and its respect for the rule of law. 'Why', the same student asked 'should I come to study in a place where I could be attacked simply because of my skin colour, or because I wear a face mask?"

The Health Secretary, Matt Hancock, deplored attacks on Chinese in UK. China's ambassador to the UK, for his part, criticised MP's for attacking China.

The virus may have originated in Wuhan but it is not a Chinese disease. None of the other pandemics which arose in other parts of the world could be attributed exclusively to those particular regions. The Zika virus epidemic appeared in South America in 2015. The virus is transmitted by mosquitoes and was first identified in bats in Zika forest in Uganda in 1974. The virus has African and Asian strains and it is related to Dengue, Japanese Encephalitis and Yellow Fever. Does one call Zika a South America disease and hold all South Americans responsible for it?

Take MERV (Middle Eastern Respiratory Virus) which originated in the Middle East. It was first reported in Saudi Arabia. Neither does one call MERV a 'Saudi Arabian' disease nor does one castigate persons of Saudi Arabian origin.

The danger of associating the disease with a particular region of the world is to add a nationalistic narrative to it. This is then a convenient springboard from which to stigmatise a nation and its population. In the globally connected world we live in, diseases can and do spread rapidly. Fifty years ago for e.g. malaria or worm infestations were relatively rare in the UK.

We in the UK have long moved away from having a stigma associated with for e.g. HIV/AIDS. Many would recall the terms ' gay virus syndrome, 'gay plague' and 'gay bug' which were used in the early 1980' to describe HIV/AIDS. There were even other stigmatising terms like GRID (gay related immune deficiency) and 'gay cancer'. These terms conveyed a sense of 'punishment' for those who were homosexual. In the yearning for a meaning of disease a prevalent view at the time was that people, 'deserved' what they got. These views arose out of ignorance. Nothing is further from the trust. As knowledge has advanced we are now wiser.

What Covid-19 has done is to lay open the racial undercurrents in society. Now, in addition to colour, religious beliefs, sexual persuasion etc, disease has become a useful racial marker to marginalise and discriminate against sections of the community.

The Australian Prime Minister Scott Morrison, spoke clearly about racism and Covid-19 when he said 'the virus started in Wuhan, in China, that's what happened, that's just a fact. But that doesn't mean that this … has any nationalistic, or any other sort of characteristics to it. That's just where it started."

In the UK, we like to think we are better than the small minority of racial bigots who would use any event or excuse to inflame racial hatred. We are, in the words of the late Martin Luther King Jr., of nearly sixty years ago, living in a nation where others 'will not be judged by the colour of their skin but by the content of their character'.

Most countries have experienced racism in some form or another related to Covid-19. Paradoxically some of the worst examples of racism are seen within China itself. People from Wuhan and Hubei are discriminated against by their Chinese compatriots. People from Wuhan have been refused hotel accommodation outside of Wuhan. Local government officials have had to locate specific hotels where people from Wuhan could be accommodated. In some cities, like in Jingxing, people were rewarded for reporting anyone coming from Wuhan. Some were paid 1000 remimbi in cash while others were rewarded with face masks.

Discrimination within China is great because of fears of second and subsequent waves of the infection. People have refused to board planes if there were persons from Wuhan on board.

Foreigners are also discriminated against for fear of them spreading the virus to Chinese. Foreigners are referred to as 'foreign trash'. A cartoon was circulated in China of people in protective gear disinfecting foreigners and throwing them in to bins. The worst excesses of racism by the Chinese are the manner in which they treat people from Africa during the Covid-19 crisis. Africans were summarily evicted from their accommodation with no alternative places provided for them to live in. There were examples of Africans being denied accommodation, attendance at hospitals etc. Some African nationals were forcibly tested for Covid-19, their passports confiscated or they were deported. The governments of Uganda, Kenya and Ghana demanded explanations of the Chinese for the latter's action against their nationals. Ghana's foreign minister, Shirley Ayorkor Botchwey 'had summoned the Chinese ambassador to express her disappointment and demand action'. In a letter of protest African ambassadors demanded that their nationals not be ejected from hotels and other accommodation, no confiscation of passports, no forced testing and arrest and no deportation of their nationals especially in Guandong. The behaviour of Chinese people in China towards others was attributed to fears of a resurgence of infection and a second wave of Covid-19. But the Chinese vice-foreign minister noted that 90% of imported cases of COVID-19 were due to Chinese nationals returning home from abroad. The initial response from China was silence, then denial and finally comments that they were taking the matter seriously.

All these reports are worrying and stand in contrast to what China expects of the rest of the world.

The comments by the Chinese ambassador in the UK and a Chinese student, who expected more draconian measures by the UK to deal with Covid-19, show the double-speak at the heart of Chinese establishment.

An important aspect of the Covid-19 crisis is the disparity in deaths in the UK between white people and those from black, Asian and minority ethnic backgrounds – called BAME in the UK. While age, sex and obesity are the most important factors that affect illness and survival from Covid-19, other features have also come to be recognised. Race and ethnicity is one set of factors that adversely affect survival. A report by Public Health England showed that people of Bangladeshi origin had twice the rate of death as those of white origin. People of other Asian origin, Pakistanis, Chinese and those from the Caribbean and other black persons had a 10-50% increased risk of dying compared to a white person. The publication of this report coincided with the race riots in the USA following the death of George Floyd in Minneapolis.

Research from University College London (UCL) showed that people from ethnic minorities are at greater risk of getting infected with Covid-19. A report showed that 35% of patients who are critically ill with Covid-19 are from BAME communities. Now this is worrying because a census in 2011 showed that only 14% of people In England and Wales are from BAME households.

In the James Bond novel 'Goldfinger', Ian Fleming wrote about Auric Goldfinger, the principal character, who said 'Mr. Bond, they have a saying in Chicago, 'Once is happenstance, twice is coincidence, the third time it is enemy action'.

For some reason I was drawn to this statement by Goldfinger when I read that the actress Miriam Margolyes had said on Channel 4 TV that she "had difficulty not wanting Boris Johnson to die". She went on to say 'I wanted him to die and then I thought that reflects badly on me and I don't want to be the sort of person who wants people to die'.

'So then I wanted him to get better, which he did do'.

'But he didn't get better as a human being and I really would prefer that.'

Appalling and ugly as this appeared at the time why did it make me think of what Goldfinger said to James Bond? And my mind raced back to what she said about David Cameron, a previous UK Prime Minister.

She was on Australian TV in January 2019 and the discussion was about Brexit. Miriam Margolyes said 'Well I'm not allowed to say the words that spring to mind because it's early in the morning.

'But I think it's a load of … bollocks is what it is. It's wrong and it's based on ignorance, people were lied to, politicians didn't tell the truth, particularly Boris Johnson and it's a disaster for England, it really is.

'I don't think it's going to end, I think it's going to go on for years and we are wasting our resources and our time and our focus. It's absolute nonsense, piffle'.

'David Cameron who was our prime minster he should be boiled in oil. It's just an absolute waste.'

So her statement about Boris Johnson was not 'happenstance or coincidence' or bad taste. This was probably her deeply held beliefs, that she wanted two UK Prime Ministers to die.

Both Prime Ministers are Conservative while Miriam Margolyes is a member of the Labour Party.

A rail union boss had sparked outrage after saying he would 'throw a party' if Boris Johnson died of coronavirus. Steve Hedley, assistant chief of The National Union of Rail, Maritime and Transport Workers said that he would throw a party if Boris Johnson died and he hoped that the whole cabinet would get Covid-19.

Earlier in April 2020 Sheila Oakes who was mayor of Heanor in Derbyshire posted a comment on Facebook saying that Boris Johnson 'completely deserves' to have coronavirus. Following this the Labour whip was withdrawn from her.

It does not come as a surprise that all three persons who spoke these words are Labour Party supporters. Mr. Chris Emmas-Williams who is head of the local Labour group in Heanor, wrote 'In no circumstances can I or the Labour Group condone this sort of behaviour, it is not in being with the standards expected in public life or office. A full investigation will take place and appropriate action will be taken in line with the Labour Party rules and regulations.'

In the case of Miriam Margolyes it was not ugly; it is bad. She thought the statement she made 'reflects badly on her'. Quite right! She was not concerned about the effect of what she said was likely to be on the Prime Minster.

She may be a role model for many children and young people after her part in Harry Potter. One shudders to think about the example that has been set.

When Mrs. Theresa May became Prime Minister of UK in July 2016 she replaced Mr. George Osborne who was Chancellor of the Exchequer at the time. George Osborne apparently told colleagues at the Evening Standard newspaper that he would not rest until Theresa May was "chopped up in bags in my freezer". When asked for his view on the comment, Mrs. May's official spokesman official spokesman said: "The contents of the former chancellor's freezer are not a matter for me."

All these words reminds one, again of 'death parties' after the death of Baroness Thatcher and chants of "Maggie, Maggie Maggie, dead, dead, dead'

Perhaps it is also worth, at this stage recalling what Ricky Gervais said when he hosted the Golden Globes Awards in 2020. *'don't use the platform to make a political speech. You're in no position to lecture the public about anything. You know nothing about the real world. Most of you spent less time in school than Greta Thunberg'.*

If we cannot disagree amicably, we are encouraging hatred and enmity. To use illness or death as a tool of vengeance is unpardonable. Lockdown is a vulnerable period for the vast majority- concerns for health, family, jobs etc. At a time like the present, when all of us need to come together to fight an unseen enemy within our ranks, there is no place for being divisive. Disagree yes, hatred no.

It is timely to reflect on the words of the late Senator John McCain of the USA. The US presidential election campaign of 2008 was between Senator McCain for the Republican Party and Barak Obama for the Democratic Party. During the election campaign a woman came up to McCain and said, 'I can't trust Obama. I have read about him, and he's not, he's not — he's an Arab.' McCain shook his head, took the microphone from the woman's hand and said, 'No ma'am; He's a decent family man, a citizen that I just happen to have disagreements with on fundamental issues, and that's what this campaign is all about.' He went on to say, 'I admire Sen. Obama and his accomplishments, I will respect him. I want everyone to be respectful, and let's make sure we are'

While Covid-19 is rampaging across the world causing suffering and death in its wake, countries and blocks appear to be acting selfishly to secure their own supply of any future vaccine against the infection.

The United States has pledged $1.2 billion to the pharmaceutical giant, Astra Zeneca, to get the first 300 million doses of a vaccine that it hoped to produce.

France, Italy and the Netherlands had apparently written to the EU Commission stating that vaccines is "one of the most urgent issues that the European Union has to address at present" Following this some countries have formed a group with the purpose of not losing out to either the United States or China in the race to get a vaccine against the coronavirus.

It was said that Europe must build up a "market power" in order to survive in the struggle for vaccines.

There is an urgent need for a vaccine. But these machinations by countries show a degree of selfishness and pursuit of advantage above the needs of human beings worldwide.

Universal availability of a vaccine for Covid-19 and indeed any vaccine is a global issue. Dr.Tedros said that countries that hoard any successful coronavirus vaccine will extend the pandemic by excluding other countries which will continue to remain susceptible to the virus. He said that there was a need to 'prevent vaccine nationalism'. After all we are all in this together is a constant reminder during the pandemic. Universal vaccine availability is the ultimate test of human altruism.

In late August we heard that private equity firms were proposing to seek government aid to help bail out firms that they had bought or in which they have a controlling stake in. It is natural for the government to help out firms in difficulty so as to save as many jobs as possible and to prevent the collapse of a company. But hedge fund firms are usually not short of cash. On the contrary they are awash with money. These are financial giants that bought out struggling firms with the aim of turning them around by making them lean and more efficient. Often what happens is the companies are loaded with debt while maximum profits are extracted from the companies they run. There has to be a different business model than the current way in which firms are bought and run by private equity firms.

Euthanasia is commonly practised on animals in the terminal stages of their lives. Many of us have experienced our beloved pets being put to rest. Euthanasia has long been a humane way of ending an animal's in the last days of its life. Another reason for considering euthanasia is when a zoo is unable to manage its animals, provide them with acceptable conditions for living and when no suitable other arrangements are available like the transfer of animals to another zoo.

With Covid-19 many, if not all, zoological gardens the world over are under escalating financial pressures. The loss of income comes arises from keeping a zoo closed and so deprived of income from visitors. One of the biggest outlays in a zoo is the cost of feeding its animals. Take away a zoo's income and its animals are immediately at risk.

Euthanasia of healthy animals is the stark choice facing many zoos. And that is not all.

The director at Neumünster Zoo in Germany has already made a list of animals they would slaughter first. The zoo is even considering feeding some animals to others as a last resort. The same sad, drastic, yet inevitable step is being considered by the Indonesian Zoo Association.

Zoo keepers at Twycross Zoo in Leicestershire, UK say that some animals, especially chimpanzees, are missing the human interaction that comes from visitors. Keepers at Moscow zoo say that pandas appear to be 'missing something' and pandas have been noted to approach any person that passes by their enclosures.

Twycross zoo is a specialist primate zoo where one can see four great apes - gorilla, orang-utan, bonobo and chimpanzee. Heart disease affects the great apes and Twycross Zoo in association with some universities has been conducting research into heart disease in these primates.

It cost £ 500,000 each month to maintain the Twycross zoo.

British zoos have drawn up contingency plans to help cope during lockdown, with aid from government. In some cases they have been sharing resources. However the longer that lockdown continues, zoos and aquaria will face unprecedented pressure which may lead to the closure of some of them.

The Department of Environment, Food and Rural Affairs would provide financial support for up to three months.

While swans returned to the canals in Venice during lockdown, animals in zoological gardens across the world face the prospect of being killed. While Venice did not want too many visitors, animals, especially apes in zoos, are missing human contact. Suddenly the phrase 'we are all in this together' assumes an entirely different and depressing new meaning.

The quiet roads during lockdown have been a bonanza for some drivers. They have chosen to use the roads and motorways as racing tracks. It was reported that two-thirds of Police forces have recorded speeding in excess of 100 miles per hour. In the first three weeks of lockdown eight drivers were caught at speeds in excess of 130 miles per hour (mph). The highest speed recorded was by a Porsche care being driven on the M1 motorway at 163 mph. Metropolitan Police said that during lockdown they had encountered a 119% increasing in speeding enforcement, while extreme speeding enforcement had gone up 181% compared to the same period in 2019. Speeding drivers put the public at risk, especially health care workers and those who work in other essential service, who were more likely to be walking or cycling to work. Also accidents are likely to be horrific at high speeds. These would need emergency services to attend with ambulance crews who would be drawn away from other life saving work related to Covid-19.

One of the most bizarre events, which went against the grain of the time, was the Adria tennis tournament stage by Novak Djokovic, the Wimbledon champion. The tournament was held in Belgrade in Serbia and Zadar in Croatia in June 2020. His views on natural remedies and his anti-vaccination opinion were already well known. But to see him and other tennis players showing no regard to social distancing in their tournament and partying in close contact with others defies description. This was at a time when there were signs of resurgence of infections in China, South Korea and Germany. When several participants including Mr. Djokovic, his wife and his fitness trainer all succumbed to the virus infection, the tournament was cancelled. This was a serious act of callousness and no apology by Mr. Djokovic afterwards to those who got the infection could compensate for the unnecessary risk that the public had been subjected to. As one commentator said of Mr. Djokovic 'enormous irresponsibility and huge immaturity. They were totally careless. It is difficult for me to find the words. I sum it up as a horror show'. Nearly half a million people across the world had died by this time from Covid-19. Many families have lost loved ones and had been left devastated.

The news that Members of Parliament (MP) were offered an extra

£10000 to help them work from home during the pandemic must come as a surprise to most people. Those who are struggling to make ends meet during lockdown would be very angry and justifiably so.

MP's are paid for office costs which are used to help support a MP's constituency office. This amounts to about £26,000 per year. The additional £10,000 is to allow MP's to work from home and can be used by them for staff salaries, heating expenses, equipment, laptops etc. It is as though these were not already available. These items are usually paid for by the normal expenses supplement that all MP's get. One MP tweeted that most of the extra £10000 will never be spent! If this is so, why was the offer made?

Schools in Singapore used video-conferencing facilities as a means of teaching and learning during lockdown. But there are downsides. While it has not happened in the UK, in Singapore the Zoom app had to be shut down when two men intruded into a geography lesson exposing their genitals and inviting girls to expose themselves.

When it seemed that there was likely to be a lockdown or some form of restrictions on life and work, there were immediate concerns in some sections of the public of shortages of food and other essentials. This was a trigger for many to rush to supermarkets and stock on various items. So it was that we encountered scenes on TV and images in newspapers of people buying more than what they needed and in reality hoarding. The phrase ' bog roll bandits' was born because shopping trolleys appeared to be so full of toilet rolls that one could not see the face of the person navigating the trolley through crowds in the supermarket aisles!. Obviously people were worried about food shortages and followed the normal human impulse to buy in excess, over and above their immediate needs. This is not an unusual occurrence. We see the same phenomenon at Christmas, Easter and before bank holidays. Often one wonders if all the food purchased would be consumed. After all, households in the UK are known to waste on average 4.5 miliion tonnes of edible food each year, worth about £14 billion. This works out at about £700 per year for an average family with children. In the world as a whole the United Nations Food and Agriculture Organisation estimates that one third of all food produced in the world is lost or wasted.

Buying more than one's needs or hoarding, apart from being wasteful, deprives others of their share of food and necessities. We saw the sad picture of a healthcare worker staring at empty shelves after her long shift at work. She and her family were deprived of food that day by those who bought more that their needs. This picture had a profound effect on many in the public. It prompted supermarkets to reserve a time when front-line workers, who were providing care during the Covid-19 crisis, could purchase their needs.

Even with dedicated time for healthcare workers and social distancing in supermarkets, there have been shortages of many items. The public were alerted to the possibility of food shortages. People tried to purchase milk and found the shelves empty of milk in supermarkets. It was therefore surprising to see a picture in the newspapers of a farmer throwing milk down the drain. This picture did not make any sense when there was obvious shortage of milk in supermarkets. Obviously there was something not quite right in the supply chain; there was milk in plenty at the production end but a dearth of milk for the customer. One milk supplier, Freshways, was charging nursing homes and care homes an increased price for dairy products. It was then reported that the company was simultaneously reducing its payments to farmers who produce milk. It was reported that the company was charging nursing homes 3p per litre more for milk while paying the farmer 2p per litre less. Therefore the company was hoping to make an additional profit of 5p on a litre of milk. Further inquiries by a newspaper also revealed that the company had not paid all of its farmers for about 2 months. One farmer who produces milk for Freshways said that the March 2020 payment to him from Freshways for milk supplied would not come to him until the middle of May. It was reported that a quarter of dairy farms may be unviable. The company, Freshways, for its part has also been under pressure during lockdown. It used to supply milk to restaurants, coffee houses, airports etc which remained shout during lockdown. It could not supply these establishments but was contractually obliged to purchase milk from producers.

Another report in newspapers was about a farmer in Kent who had to pour away 10,000 litres of milk as it was not collected from the farm by the milk processors. The milk processor in turn had difficulty in getting drivers during lockdown.

While all this was happening farmers had to pay their bills forcing some them into debt. In the current context it is interesting to recall that in 1996 the then Deputy Prime Minister, Michael Heseltine (now Lord Heseltine), claimed that he delayed paying his creditors to save his business from 'going bust'. This was at a time when the government of the day was encouraging firms to pay their bills in time. But he eventually paid all his creditors and apparently felt good for doing so. John Prescott, the then deputy leader of the Labour Party, accused Mr Heseltine of acting in a way which "wrecks people's lives".

A different story was seen in the case of British beef. Since the virus crisis there was reported to be a 150% increase in demand for red meats in supermarkets. Like in the case of milk there were problems in the supply chain of red meats- getting animals to abattoir and the loss of markets like restaurants, farmer's markets etc. Like milk there may have been a problem with getting meat from producers to market due to staff shortages and social distancing rules. The beef shortage prompted some supermarkets to import and display Polish minced beef on their shelves. Mince appeared to be in demand, probably for use at home in burgers. Following an outcry from meat producers, the supplies of foreign beef were withdrawn.

Supermarkets increased prices of some goods during the lockdown. One supermarket was found to have increased prices by 16%. Customers threatened to boycott the supermarket Special offers had also been withdrawn by supermarkets. By 24th April 2020 the Competition and Markets Authority had received 21,000 complaints from customers. The CMA had written to 187 companies about prices.

Banks that were encouraged to support small business following lockdown were initially slow to respond. The Governor of the Central Bank, Andrew Bailey, said that not enough had been done by banks by the third quarter of April 2020. For example only £ 2 billion had been lent under the government's coronavirus business interruption scheme. This was in contrast to the situation in for e.g. Switzerland or Germany. In Germany, financial support was immediately made available to small businesses. They were able to access cheap loans directly from banks. The rules relating to turnover thresholds of small businesses were relaxed. Banks, like Deutsche Bank, worked to try and avoid bottlenecks in the processes of delivering support to customers.

Similar rapid financial support was provided by Switzerland's Federal

Council. It provided funds to help bridge liquidity shortfalls to over 75,000 businesses early in lockdown, which was introduced on 16th March.

For UK banks to claim that they cannot deal with the huge demand for assistance does not explain the hold up, when other countries have managed to act quickly in helping businesses. Assessing risks, coping with demand, dealing with bank staff working from home, social distancing etc are common to all countries during this crisis.

The events during and following the banking crisis of 2008 must be a painful worry to businesses and especially smaller ones. Then in 2008 banks treated their business customers appallingly by charging high fees, disposing of business assets and bankrupting individuals. Banks would not want to be seen to be acting in a similar manner during the Covid-19 pandemic. It is now incumbent on the Governor of the Central Bank to ensure that the business loan scheme is easier to access, is fair and helps, especially small businesses,

At that time of the banking crisis of 2008, Royal Bank of Scotland was claimed to have "harmed their customers through their decisions and caused their financial downfall'. Struggling firms were passed on to a division in the bank called Global Restructuring group. Exorbitant fees charged by GRG caused some businesses to collapse. Following collapse assets of the business were acquired by GRG, which then proceeded to dispose of them. The Financial Conduct Authority (FCA) said at the time that it did not have the power to investigate the activities of GRG. Why the FCA could not investigate and act on obvious financial misconduct is surprising to say the least. It is somewhat lame and of no relief to those who suffered for the FCA to claim that it could not act outside its remit. What was its remit if it could not investigate financial misconduct? The current Governor for the Bank of England, Andrew Bailey, was the Chairman of the FCA from January 2016. He said of GRG 'it is important for all who work in this sector to regain the public's trust. I must acknowledge the distress felt by many of GRG's customers. The firm's relations with its customers were often insensitive, dismissive and sometimes too aggressive; these failings made an already stressful situation worse'.

Now in 2020 many businesses are facing an even worse situation, where survival after lockdown must surely be at risk. Many owners of small businesses may be facing collapse and even bankruptcy. There could not be a better time for the banking industry in the UK to work for local communities and for the benefit of the economy. In so doing it may take the first tentative steps in regaining public trust and in rehabilitating itself.

Banks were reminded that the public bailed many of them out in 2008.

The actions of some companies that have used the government's furlough scheme for employees. drew much attention in newspapers. The furlough scheme allowed companies to set aside their employees during lockdown without loss of their jobs. The government agreed to pay 80% of n employees wage up to a ceiling of £2500 per person per month. In this way companies could retain their employees and not lose skills. Personnel and skills would be important after lockdown when it is hoped that companies could return to their usual work levels. But many in the public asked why some rich company owners could not pay their employees without using the furlough scheme.

Almost 7.5 million workers from about 1 million businesses are on the scheme at the time of this writing.

Virgin Atlantic airlines have placed 8000 of the airlines employees in the scheme. He had been criticized for not using his wealth to avoid furlough. He has sought £500 million from the UK government to help save the airline. Sir Richard Branson who owns Virgin Atlantic apparently even pledged his Caribbean island, Necker Island, as collateral but this appears to have been rejected by the government. In the USA Virgin Atlantic filed for bankruptcy as a means of protecting the airline and its assets in USA. Mike Ashley who owned Newcastle United Football Club and owner of the Frasers Group has placed the majority of his 18,000 staff in the furlough scheme. Sir Philip Green placed 14,500 of staff in his Arcadia Group on furlough. Liverpool Football Club placed 200 of their non-playing staff on furlough. This led to criticism from supporters and players especially as the club had just announced pre-tax profits of £ 42 million. Liverpool is the world's seventh richest football club. This had the effect of probably strengthening Tottenham Hotspur supporters to pressure their club, Tottenham Hotspur Football Club in north London to do the same. Tottenham Hotspur reversed their decision. Easyjet sent 7000 of its staff on furlough but it still paid a dividend totalling £174 million to its shareholders. Easyjet is cutting 4500 jobs which is about a third of its workforce. Job losses of 3000 each were seen in Virgin Atlantic and Ryanair. There is no doubt that the airline industry is severely affected by the pandemic and lockdown. It is also uncertain when any reasonable level of activity will return to the airline sector. However, one wonders if some of the profits and cash reserves that these businesses have, could not be used instead of seeking help from the government job retention scheme.

Victoria Beckham and her husband, David, are together worth in the region of £350 million. Mrs. Beckham initially applied for money from the government furlough scheme for 30 of her staff of 120. Facing public criticism she withdrew the application for furlough funds.

The actions of some of the business leaders in the country showed the disparity between the haves and the have not's of society. It is perfectly acceptable for millionaire and billionaire businessmen to avail themselves and their businesses of the government's furlough scheme for their employees. However to many in the public this may not sit well with the apparent ease with which they appeared to walk away from their businesses while expecting the taxpayer to help out. It is often forgotten that the profits of the wealthy are generated by the work of their employees. Compare these activities with the furlough of Prince Charles's staff. About 200 staff at The Princes Foundation was sent on furlough with Prince Charles paying the wage bill of about £ 4.5 million, without resorting to the Exchequer.

British Airways was taken to task by MP's who accused it of being a 'national disgrace'. It was accused of using the Covid-19 crisis to cut 12,000 jobs in the airline. BA was in receipt of £35 million to help with staff wages. MP's were concerned that despite receipt of money from the governments' job retention scheme, it was planning to make large numbers of its staff redundant. MP's suggested that the government change the rules to prevent a company from laying off staff while it was in receipt of government help to retain staff. However the furlough scheme provided some companies and their staff a 'breathing space' to permit any previously planned review and redundancy scheme. This allowed some employees, who would anyway have been made redundant, to be in receipt of some wages for a few more months.

Another notable example is Sir James Dyson who had not used the furlough scheme for his employees.

Could some of the businesses that sought refuge in the government's furlough scheme be examples of the unacceptable face of capitalism?

Airline passengers whose flights could not be completed or which were cancelled due to lockdown face a long period of uncertainty before they get refunds of the monies that they had paid. European Union law is clear and states that passengers should get their money back within seven days. There is no obligation for passengers to accept vouchers instead of a full refund of money paid. But it appears that some airlines are exerting pressure on passengers to accept vouchers instead of money. Easyjet for example is said to have saved £700 million by encouraging customers to accept vouchers instead of it having to pay out the money. It re-introduced the refund claim form to its website after protests.

Ryanair had said that customers have the options of either a voucher or refund of their money. Vouchers can be exchanged for cash after 12 months if they have chosen not to fly. But it warned customers that moneys would be paid into their accounts only after the current Covid-19 crisis had settled. It said it has to deal with 10,000 times the usual volume of cancellations.

To be fair to the airlines it must be said that, at the times the rules were written, there was probably no thought of large scale interruptions to flights of the kind we have witnessed in these unprecedented times. Most airlines would have had a relatively small number of staff to deal with cancellations and claims for refunds. A crisis of the current magnitude was unlikely to have been imagined, especially with staff being absent from their desks and working from home. It is therefore to some extent understandable that there is delay in processing requests for refunds and for customers seeing the money in tier bank accounts.

Some airlines have not helped the situation by appearing to be tardy in dealing with the volume of work. For example more telephone lines would have helped to some extent. Also it is known that some airlines have information in small print to the effect that those who chose to change their booked holiday for a cash refund would have to pay an administration fee of up to £200. This amount cannot be justified by the work involved in making a refund.

Sir Stelios Haji-Ioannou, founder of Easy jet said that accepting vouchers is a risk, as customers might lose all their money if the airline collapsed. In this event vouchers would have no value whatsoever.

Not only airlines but also other holiday firms have been reluctant to refund customers who had booked prior to lockdown. One such firm was Hoseasons which was reported by customers to the Competition and Markets Authority (CMA) for not making refund of payments to customers. The CMA had set up a special Covid-19 task force which had received about 4500 complains about UK holiday companies.

Travel insurers in the UK have also been reluctant to pay for cancelled holidays. Direct Line insurance company advised those who booked travel insurance with a credit card to seek refunds from their card-issuing banks first, before approaching the company. The FCA said that insurers should not be advising customers to first seek reimbursement from the card issuer. However the FCA has not shown itself to be effective in enforcing its view.

Andrea Coscelli, Chief Executive of the CMA said 'we know the pandemic is presenting businesses with challenges too, but it's not right that people are being left hundreds or even thousands of pounds out of pocket – on top of having to sacrifice their holidays."Consumer protection law exists for a reason; businesses must observe the law or face the possibility of enforcement action.'

In June 2020 BA, EasyJet, and Ryanair brought High Court action with the purpose of challenging the government's decision to impose a 14 day quarantine of passengers coming from abroad. These three companies claimed that there is no scientific evidence to support quarantine while at the same time claiming that the rules are too stringent. The average traveller is an interested party in this matter and would like to know what scientific evidence to the contrary the airlines have. And what is meant by the claim that the 14-day quarantine is too stringent? This is a matter of great public interest and it is only right that any information is readily available for scrutiny. Who would be responsible if a court scrapped the 14-day quarantine and there followed a spike in infection? Prudence requires that every reasonable precaution be taken to limit second and subsequent spikes in infection. "Those who forget history are condemned to repeat it" is attributed to the American philosopher George Santayana. In the Spanish flu of 1918 there was a second and even a third spike in infection that contributed to the enormous numbers who died.

There were claims that the Police in different areas appear to have interpreted the guidance about lockdown in different ways. There was a threat in Northamptonshire of customers shopping trolleys and shopping baskets being checked! What, one wonders, were they looking for in the fight against coronavirus?

In early May 2020 South Yorkshire Police offered an apology after posting on its website "between essential saunter in jeans as exercise, an essential trip to the shops for egg custards and essential trip to the cash machine for £20 to use in the morning, we've offered a lot of advice." The same Police had told a person in Rotherham that he could not use his front garden during lockdown!

It was equally hilarious to read the story of a man mowing his friend's lawn being questioned by Police. He could claim he was exercising while helping his friend and maintaining a social distance!

Reports from Police across the country reveal the extent to which people have stretched the meaning of the phrase 'essential travel' . A person was caught travelling from Edinburgh to Wigan to buy a puppy. A father and his son were stopped by police for driving around hunting for Pokémon. Some of the interpretations of 'essential' are nothing short of hilarious. Sports Direct, the sportswear company, remained open at the onset of lockdown claiming that it was "uniquely well placed to help keep the UK as fit and healthy as possible". Cabinet Minister, Michael Gove replied "People can walk, run or cycle, they should, but there is no reason for a store like Sports Direct to remain open." Sports Direct closed its doors.

By the end of April 2020 more than 9000 fines had been issued by Police in England and Wales to people for breaching lockdown restrictions

A poll showed that 75% of the public supported the Police in their ensuring that the rules on social distancing were followed. But a third of those polled thought that Police were too strict.

Insurers have not always been acting in a sympathetic way towards individuals and businesses. Businesses usually take out insurance to cover interruptions to the businesses which cause loss of revenue. That is the sole reason for paying out insurance premiums to cover this eventuality. Of course not all insurance policies would have provided this type of cover. However, if business interruption was covered by a policy it would be expected that an insurance company would pay out when a relevant claim is made. Business interruption claims are likely to cost insurers close to £ 1 billion. In Switzerland the insurer Helvetia had agreed to pay out while in Bavaria some insurers had agreed to pay a part of the losses incurred by hotels and restaurants that are not in receipt of state aid. A group of businesses wrote to the Association of British Insurers (ABI) claiming that their businesses with relevant cover, and for which they had paid the premiums, had not had positive responses from their insurers. At the time of writing the outcome of any legal action is awaited but it is understandable if insurance companies refuse to pay out for circumstances that were not covered when insurance was purchased. Covid-19 is an unexpected event and how it would be interpreted in law in the light of the wording of insurance policies would not doubt have ramifications beyond the pandemic.

In response to growing concern about the matter the Financial Conduct Authority (FCA) issued a statement to the effect that it is seeking court adjudication on the contractual obligation between the insured and insurance companies on the matter. This would help to resolve the issue and would be fair to both the insured and insurance accompanies. FCA has advised insurance companies to act promptly in settling these claims and where appropriate to make interim payments. It is interesting and concerning to note that FCA recognises that the wording of policies vary between insurance companies. Whatever the wording in a policy, the average business person would have paid a premium for business interruption in the hope that all interruptions to a business would be covered. Some policies may have excluded war, terrorism and 'acts of god', whatever the latter may mean. At the time of taking out a policy, business interruption due to a pandemic may not have been anticipated and therefore likely not to have been included in the insurance policy. One can imagine insurance companies invoking the concept of an 'act of god' to relieve them from the obligation to pay out. The lawyer Steve Myers (Sir Billy Connolly) in the film 'The Man Who Sued God' was able to convince the judge in the case that the phrase 'act of god' is misleading. So also it is in this instance. But as Sam Woods, Deputy Governor of the Bank of England said ' it doesn't make sense to expect insurance companies to cover huge things they had no expectation of covering. They would not expect to cover a very wide pandemic-driven business interruption. They deliberately excluded that because they could see it would be a very large hit.' The estimated cost of claims is likely to be in the region of £1 billion. Here lies a dilemma- some insurers could collapse if they had to meet this bill for business interruption while on the other hand businesses could collapse if there is no financial help forthcoming soon. The government could step in to help develop a scheme to deal with such matters. Following the pandemic it is very likely that most, if not all, insurers would justifiably exclude pandemics and the like from being covered.

Government issued guidance to landlords and tenants on how to proceed during the Covid-19 crisis period. Under the Coronavirus Act 2020 landlords would not be able to commence eviction proceedings unless they have given their tenants three months notice. The law courts in UK also suspended housing possession cases for three months. Government appealed to tenants and landlords to work together during this period. Tenants were advised to continue to pay rent. If they were having difficulty in paying rent, they were advised to discuss the problem early with their landlords.

The Lord Chief Justice has advised judges to be mindful of their judgements and their likely effects on public health. As such court proceeding about repossessions would be suspended as a matter of priority. The same advice would apply to lodgers. This was an important piece of the Coronavirus Act. Any eviction would place the people affected not only at risk of homelessness but also at risk o getting and spreading Covid-19. The Housing Ombudsman Service has provided useful information to landlords. Landlords, by and large, have responded fairly during lockdown and have acted sympathetically to tenants.

Asylum seekers are in a very difficult position during lockdown. Asylum seekers need to submit their claim for asylum at the Home Office in London. This is difficult to accomplish during lockdown and especially with social distancing rules in force. At the same time it is reported that the Home Office is unable to process applications for asylum until lockdown has been lifted. The Home Office says that asylum seekers who have nowhere to live and are therefore destitute, would be helped by its department in Croydon, South London.

Some asylum seekers are in detention centres awaiting deportation.

Other asylum seekers need to report regularly to the Home office. With lockdown, regular reporting has been temporarily suspended. This has come as an enormous relief to this group of asylum seekers. The UK is said to have a 'hostile environment' approach to asylum seekers. Having to report regularly is an alarming experience for most asylum seekers. Some say they spend several sleepless nights worrying about the day they have to report. They often find reporting an intimidating experience and many suffer anxiety related to it. Charities hope that there would be a re-think on how the government deals with asylum seekers after lockdown.

Another problems facing asylum seekers is having to choose between food and medicine. The weekly allowance for an asylum seeker is about £35. There are additional financial supplements if an asylum seeker is a child, or is pregnant etc. But the total amount barely meets the needs of the person for living expenses, excluding housing and utility bills, for a week. Also with shortages in shops during lockdown, many have to pay more than the usual prices to obtain essential items as they struggle to provide for their families during this period. The cost of a television, mobile telephones, toys for children etc have to be met with this small allowance. A mobile phone is not a luxury. It is a necessity to help keeping in touch with family and friends in a new and strange country.

Not all people have benefitted from the support schemes that are available during lockdown. The free school meal voucher is an important example. The voucher is worth £15 per child per week. Parents can spend this money in supermarkets for food. Schools have had difficulty operating the system on line and not all households have internet access. Also the vouchers cannot be used in all the supermarkets that parents could use. For e.g., Aldi and Lidl supermarkets were not initially on the list where vouchers may be used. Parents avoid Waitrose and Marks and Spencer's due to cost. When one is shopping on a limited budget, one has to be economical with shopping. Most parents know of and experience the difficulty of juggling with money and needs during every shopping trip for the family.

There is also a stigma attached to vouchers which many parents are conscious of. A change to a cash based system would remove the stigma while providing greater flexibility, like using the corner shop in an emergency.

The Office of National Statistics found a link between household income and availability of internet access. In households where the income was between £6000 and £10,000, only 50% had internet access. Households where the income was in excess of £40,000 had near 100% internet access. Internet poverty is a significant domestic and social disability. It affects access to educational material for children. The internet is nowadays the equivalent of textbooks. Take away the internet and one has taken away a child's learning material. No meaningful or productive learning can occur without access to information on the internet. Likewise some schools have provided learning material on the internet during lockdown. The child without access to the internet is immediately at a disadvantage. This in turn works through into poor education achievement, even without Covid-19 and lockdown.

The attitude of some university vice-chancellors must surely come out top in any such league of ugliness related to Covid-19. While staff at these institutions of learning has been furloughed, some vice-chancellors have continued to benefit from their hugely inflated salaries. Take for e.g. the vice chancellor of the University of Bolton who earns a salary of £290,000 per annum. The university is ranked 125th out of 131 in a league table of universities. Or the vice chancellor of Oxford University who refused a pay cut from a salary of £425,000 per year. How can such enormous salaries be justified when the universities are collectively in debt to the tune of about £10 billion! One cannot escape the conclusion that some of these universities had jettisoned, some time ago, the principle that they are seats of learning and enlightenment. Rather they are now run as businesses, attracting more custom in the form of students. In return some of the degrees attained by students do not always prepare them for the workplace. Prospective employers would say that graduates are often not adequately equipped for the work that is eventually expected of them.

It is known that Cambridge University was seeking financial assistance from the Government. One is surprised when one hears about this as the University has financial reserves of about £5billion. At a time when most small businesses and households are struggling, it is scandalous that a rich institution seeks taxpayer's money. It would be advised to reflect on its role in the country at a time of crisis?

What Adam Smith wrote over two hundred years ago is appropriate today as it was then "In the university of Oxford, the greater part of the public professors have, for these many years, given up altogether even the pretence of teaching'. This is as true today as it ever was when one hears that senior academics and professors spend time at international conferences with little in the way of leadership in their departments and institutions. Universities have become big businesses with their prime activity being income generation. Academic freedom is lost and the culture of learning and healthy debate diluted or in many instances eliminated. Freedom of speech, the bedrock of our democracy has currently no place in some universities. Academic debate and rigour has been sacrificed at the altar of political correctness and money.

Take the case of the previous dictator of Libya, the late Colonel Muammar Gaddaffi. The Gaddaffi Foundation pledged to donate £1.5 million for research at the London School of Economics. When Colonel Gaddaffi spoke to the school via video link, he was referred to as 'Brother Leader'. Gaddafi's son, Saif Gaddaffi was awarded a PhD for which he wrote a thesis which many suspect was plagiarised or ghost-written. The Director of the LSE, Sir Howard Davis, resigned following the Libyan Civil war and the allegations of irregularities. Roger Cohen wrote in The New York Times 'It may be possible to sink to greater depths but right now I can't think how. ... How did we back, use and encourage the brutality of Arab dictators over so many years?...'

The same question may be asked now.

Covid-19 is a good time to look at what place universities serve in society. Universities need to return urgently to being places of learning, academic freedom, uninhibited inquiry and research. The word *university* is from the Latin 'uni*versitas magistrorum et scholarium*, meaning a "community of teachers and scholars". Universities should not been seen as degree factories. Also they need to do away with banning of speakers and platforming; allow ideas to be discussed and where needed defeated by the force of argument and reasoning. In so doing we would encourage those 'snowflakes' among our student population to develop the habit of healthy inquiry, acceptance that others may have opposing views and to inculcate in all a sense of tolerance and compromise. Society needs nothing less. One particular area of increasing concern is students with political affiliations to their own country. They are often known to stifle healthy debate, if this conflicts with their views.

In this regard it is important to note the influence Chinese students have on UK universities. Warwick University has a Chinese Students and Scholars Association (CSSA) which is affiliated to the Chinese embassy in the UK and is not part of the student's union at Warwick. CSSA is apparently in existence to look after Chinese students in universities in the UK. It monitors the activities of students and may be seen as a coercive organisation used to ensure that Chinese students virtually toe the line. Free thinking and debate are frowned upon. Therefore it influences any discussion on sensitive topics. For e.g. CSA was able to defeat a motion in Warwick University supporting democracy and free speech in Hong Kong. Students used by China to enforce its views should ideally be removed from universities. For its part China has tried to blackmail universities by threatening to withdraw students who are fee paying. This is again a form of intimidation which is all too common in China's dealings with the rest of the world. This threat shows how the CCP uses its students as an instrument of policy. If education was paramount, the CCP would not place the future of its youth at risk.

This is as good a time as any to ask whether the UK needs as many universities as it currently has. And do they need to run as businesses generating income? Does the UK need to produce or to have as many graduates? This is a good time to ask what the purpose of graduates is in society. The fundamental purpose of any education, academic, university –based or vocational, is to produce young people are who are equipped for the roles they want to have in life, for the jobs they want to do. It is of little use to have a graduate in carpentry, when good vocational training would do! Likewise there is little need for a nurse with a degree who has lost her sense of caring and vocation. In 2013 the former Labour MP, Ann Clwyd wrote of nurses who were ignoring desperately ill patients. She described one case where a nurse told the husband of a patient - 'I'm a graduate. I don't do sick'. It is time for government to allow those universities that are financially unviable or not producing the kind of graduates that the economy needs to fold. None of this implies that youngsters should be denied the chance of going to university. Often a university degree leads to disappointment, disillusionment and debt.

Schools and society need to inculcate in students the desire to seek the best way of achieving their ambitions; not all would be served well by going to university.

For any parent to hear their child being described as 'mucky, cry and wipe their snot on your trousers or on your dress' must be distressing and they would not be faulted for finding the remarks offensive. One is tempted to ask what any such teacher was expecting their charges to be. These are often little children who are vulnerable and dependent on teachers as they are on their parents and carers. They need teaching, not only of approved subjects but also social skills. They need help in their times of need when in class. Perhaps such teachers have forgotten that they are 'in loco parentis' when children are in their care. They, like the majority of caring teachers, substitute for parents when children are in class.

Fortunately the majority of teachers are devoted to their profession and find it their vocation in life. They do not see children in the same manner as described above. And they continue to worry about how lockdown has affected their children. The future of our children is at stake here. The longer their return to school is delayed the more the adverse long term effect on education and achievement in later life. Unfortunately those children from lower income families are likely to suffer most from a prolonged lockdown. The concerns of teachers and their unions about spreading infection are legitimate. But this has to be tempered with the knowledge that a zero infection risk is never likely to be achieved. When the risk of infection has reduced, as it has, it is sensible to consider a staged return to school. We do not know what the lowest safe level of infection would be for any activity, be it opening schools or going to a supermarket.

It is unfortunate that the British Medical Association (BMA) claimed that schools should not open, without providing any information in support of this claim. Fortunately it soon reversed its position. At a time like this, surrounded by concern and fear, it would be useful if responsible organizations and opinion leaders refrain from making statements in the absence of evidence to support of their views. The BMA eventually concluded that schools could open even before the 1st of June 2020.

A paper was published in the paediatric journal, Acta Paediatrica in May 2020 by Jonas Ludvigsson and colleagues. They reviewed over 700 scientific papers about children with Covid-19. They came to the conclusion that children are 'unlikely to be the main drivers of the pandemic. Opening up schools and kindergartens is unlikely to impact Covid-19 mortality rates in older people.' There has not been any outbreak of the infection in Swedish schools. At the time of writing French, German, Danish and Dutch children were back at school. The chief scientist at the WHO, Dr. Soumya Swaminathan said that children are at low risk of getting the disease, if they get it, it is milder than in adults and that they are less capable of spreading the infection to others. This does not mean that the elderly and those with another relevant medical condition should be exposed to children. But the majority of adults in school are apparently young and healthy. Teachers unions which were clamoring for evidence to support a return to school of their members now have sufficient reassurance to do so.

On Tuesday 5th May 2019 Professor Neil Ferguson resigned from SAGE due his breach of social distancing rules. Remember, he was the architect of the policy of lockdown. His mathematical modelling of risks to the UK from Covid-19 concluded that there could be about 250,000 deaths if lockdown was not implemented.

Prof. Ferguson is an epidemiologist at University College London. He has a long history of modelling in epidemiology going back to the BSE ('mad cow disease') episode, hand, foot and mouth disease in 2001 and swine flu in 2009. What an epidemiologist does is to collect information about epidemics, their infectivity and try to project the impact of a future epidemic or pandemic on a population. It is not an exact science nor is it guesswork. An epidemiologist uses a number of factors and the history of previous epidemics to predict the extent of an emerging infection. Often there is no past experience to help in calculations and predictions. For e.g. there was no previous swine flu epidemic before 2009. They use information about the nature of the virus and data collected as the infection is spreading to help predict what is likely to happen. It is therefore no wonder that they could be wrong in their prediction but they provide information about a worst case scenario. This helped them predict the likely death rate from Covid-19 if lockdown was not put in place.

He, with other scientists, persuaded government to act urgently and bring in lockdown, which it did on 23rd of March. However his partner visited him at his home on 30th March. She then made a second trip to his residence on 8th April although she thought her own husband had symptoms of Covid-19.

Prof. Ferguson said: "I accept I made an error of judgement and took the wrong course of action," and "I deeply regret any undermining of the clear messages around the continued need for social distancing."

He had done a significant amount of work for the UK, worldwide and for the WHO. His error does not undermine or reduce in any way the importance of his contributions to public health generally and in the UK's response to the pandemic.

The Health Secretary, Matt Hancock, was of the view that Prof Ferguson should have been prosecuted for being in violation of the lockdown regulations.

The Housing, Communities and Local Government Secretary Mr. Robert Jenrick travelled 150 miles from London to his home in Herefordshire. He was also seen having visited his parents in Shropshire.

Dr. Catherine Calderwood, Chief Medical Officer in Scotland was found to have broken lockdown regulations and travelled to a second home. She resigned and said she was disappointed with her behaviour "having worked so hard on the government's response" to the virus.

When lockdown came into effect on 23rd March people were advised to stay in their primary residences and not to visit second homes or holiday homes. Robert Jenrick had visited his parents' home in Shropshire. He considered his primary home to be in Herefordshire. Mr. Jenrick explained that he visited his parents to deliver essentials including medicines. He had said that by staying at home 'we protect the NHS and help save lives' and in March wrote that people need to 'make big sacrifices- especially today, on Mother's Day'.

Again the errors of these persons do not in any way diminish the work they've done or the contributions they have made in the battle against Covid-19.

Some would say these acts amount to the operation of double standards in those who should have known better. What is unfortunate is that these are opinion formers and leaders whom the average person, 'the man on the Clapham omnibus', looks to for guidance. When the guidance involves safety and the matter of life and death it seem perverse for the guidance or rules to be broken by those who want them followed by everyone for the good of all.

Separated from loved ones, unable to visit parents and grandparents, grandparents not being able to see their grandchildren etc are some of the situations all have had to endure during lockdown. The grief of parting with a loved one or not to be present at a funeral must be unimaginable. In some cases people have lost more than one member of the family to Covid-19. And still they stayed within the guidelines of lockdown.

It is illuminating to compare these events with the resignation of Don Harwin, the Arts Minister of New South Wales, Australia, who was caught by police after leaving his home. Or the New Zealand's health minister who was demoted by the Prime Minster Jacinda Arden after breaking social distancing rules. Mr. David Clark offered his resignation but she stopped short of sacking him to avoid disruption of the vital work that was being done to contain Covid-19. This is Jacinda Arden when she placed the country in lockdown "I say to all New Zealanders: the government will do all it can to protect you. Now I'm asking you to do everything you can to protect all of us. Kiwis – go home." Many across the globe praised her for her decisiveness. So highly held is she that New Zealanders even offered to loan her out! Perhaps some world leaders could avail of her services if only to appreciate the importance of 'oneness' and the value of taking people with you when you are leading. While planning the exit from lockdown she referred to the population as 'our team of five million'.

The Belgian prince, Joachim, was fined €10,400 (£9,300) in May 2020 for not adhering to the 14-day quarantine rules when he arrived in Cordoba, in the Andalusia region of Spain. He was found to have gone to a party with twenty-seven people on 26th May. What was worrying was that he tested positive for Covid-19 after the party. If he pays the fine in 15 days the amount owed would be halved. Joachim is the nephew of King Philippe of Belgium.

Many others have fallen foul of regulations brought in during the Covid-19 period. Pablo Iglesias, vice President of Spain, Leo Varadkar of Ireland and Polish Prime Minister, Mateusz Morawiecki, have had to explain themselves.

Rules are there to be followed by all. Again in New Zealand Jacinda

Arden and her partner were refused entry into a restaurant because of social distancing rules.

The story about Dominic Cummings, the Prime Minister's advisor, was extensively covered by newspapers and TV. He had driven with his wife and child from London to see his parents in Durham in north-east England, a distance of about 250 miles. He had also driven for about 30 minutes from his parent's home to Barnard Castle apparently to see if he 'could drive safely'.

A letter sent by 26 senior UK academics and health administrators to Downing Street complained about the impact of the Dominic Cummings controversy. In answer to a question at the briefing about Dominic Cummings, Professor Van-Tam said: 'In my opinion the rules are clear and they have always been clear. In my opinion they are for the benefit of all. "In my opinion they apply to all.'

The failure of the government to enforce the regulations may have contributed later on to significant breaches following which the Police turned a literal blind eye. The Black Lives Matter marches, the mass of people enjoying the day on beaches, the partying by fans of Liverpool Football Club etc showed that lockdown regulations could not be enforced. This is a significant dereliction of leadership which placed the entire population at risk.

Quarantine rules in UK carry a warning that if broken 'may' result in a fine. The word 'may' implies that rules are difficult to enforce or would not be enforced. Laws are there as much to be complied with as to be enforced. If they cannot be enforced then it becomes bad law. If other counties around the world are able to enforce rules related to lockdown, it is justifiable to ask why they cannot be enforced in the UK. Why are penalties not imposed? If there is a loophole in the law, it becomes like driving offences; they can be circumvented and they would be circumvented. The celebrity lawyer, Nick Freeman, also referred to as 'Mr. Loophole' by the press, has successfully challenged the law in relation to driving offences. This is another example where sentencing magistrates and judges are lax in interpreting and in enforcing the law. Persons flying into the UK need to be in quarantine for 14 days or they would have to pay a fine of £1,000. It was recorded that in one week the penalty was not imposed on a single passenger. It may be that all passengers were dutifully complying with the requirement to self- quarantine. Or is this another example where the authorities are unable to enforce the law?

Everyone was required to wear face masks in public from 15th June 2020 or face a penalty of £100. However guidance to rail companies is to impose the fine only as a last resort. Staff was encouraged to employ the five-E's – engage, explain, encourage, enable and enforce'. When therefore does one impose the fine? Does one impose a fine on the 5th person the Police encounter – after having engaged, encouraged, explained and enabled the preceding four persons who were not using mask? There has been an information campaign and most know about the need to wear a mask. The Mayor of London, Sadiq Kahn, called for the compulsory wearing of face masks some months ago. There are far too many examples of laxity. If one is asked to wear a mask, one should comply or face the consequences.

Kings and commoners may break rules but all have to be held to account irrespective of station. This would reinforce the message that as far as Covid-19 is concerned 'we are all in this together', as the public is constantly reminded of.

Quis custodiet ipsos custodes? wrote Juvenal, a Roman poet. Translated it reads "Who will guard the guards themselves?" and was quoted by Plato in his book 'Republic'. We judge our leaders but do not expect them to be saints. They are a microcosm of the society from which they arise. In other words, they are us with all human failings and therefore range from those with absolute altruism to psychopaths. But when the message is also about my safety and that of my family I would expect everyone else to play by the same rules. Even if they are the rule makers or rulers.

Leadership by example is more than doing what you said. The person who advises, needs to believe in what is said; he needs to buy into the message and take ownership of it. In other words they are also recipients of the message that they themselves are giving out. They must be convinced by the message and be prepared to live by it.

Leaders and opinion formers must not only 'talk the talk' but also 'walk the walk'. Many of us may have experienced people who say one thing and do another. Nothing is more destructive to morale than to see those who tell us and direct us and guide us, not abiding by what they say. Enthusiasm to comply is lost. When one sees a person who practices what he is preaching, curiosity is aroused. Even if you are disbeliever it makes you want to stop and think. Take the example of Mahatma Gandhi who committed his life to non-violent protest and took India to the promised land of independence from the British Raj. Or take the example of Nelson Mandela who upon release from prison preached reconciliation. He invited his former prison guards to his inauguration as President of South Africa. He also met with Betsie Verwoerd, widow of Hendrik Verwoerd, who was President of South Africa and who had implemented apartheid.

Lockdown is, in many ways, an experiment which has never been done in peacetime and where the public are asked to remain incarcerated in their homes. Since World War two there has been relative peace and a flowering of our freedoms. The single most important driver for the change that was asked of the population was a convincing message delivered without invoking undue fear and should reach out to seek the consent of the people. This needed the message to be given with conviction and vigour. We are all in this together, we are constantly told. But are we, if some in authority act independent of the prevailing wisdom? If the message is so lax that it has as many interpretations as there are people to whom it applies then it is not an effective message. Leaders who bend or break rules, immediately display hypocrisy. The unfortunate effect of hypocrisy is to dilute the message and invite at best, limited compliance with what is being asked of the public.

As Stephen Reicher said ' if adherence is all about a sense of 'us' then it is fatally undermined if you create a sense of 'us and them' and one of the best ways to do that is to give a sense that the government and government figures abide by a different set of rules to the public – one law for us and one law for them. It immediately creates this 'us and them' thinking and you've therefore undermined compliance'. These words are relevant to the breach of lockdown by the Prime Minister's advisor, Dominic Cummings. In Reicher's view respect for the public, equality of treatment, consistency and being in it together were all 'trashed'.

People's confidence in their government's handling of the Covid-19 crisis has dropped. Kantar is a world-wide company involved in data analysis. Research in the Group of Seven (G7) countries showed that only 48% of those who responded said that they approved of how their government managed the pandemic. The figure was 54% in March at the outset of the crisis. The UK was worst in the ratings having dropped to 33%. It was 51 % in April. Loss of trust may have contributed to the diminished confidence that people have in how the government in the UK is managing the pandemic. Events, like that involving Dominic Cumming do not help and may have contributed to a negative 'Cummings Factor'.

Trust has been a big casualty in this saga. However compelling a future message is, the loss of trust may adversely impact on its acceptance by the public. Therein lies danger for all, public and politicians, as we collectively work and contribute to suppress the virus.

o0:0o

RELEASE

About the end of May 2020 a seventy year old man was in a shopping precinct singing 'Please release me', pleading for an early exit from lockdown. After his rendition, he told those assembled and who cared to listen that he had had enough of staying at home and being prevented by his two daughters from leaving home. He was fit, able, but had heart disease and high blood pressure and was forbidden to leave the house. All his food and medicine was delivered by his caring daughters. Those readers of a certain vintage may recall this song being belted out by that ageless crooner, Engelbert Humperdinck in the 1970's and 1980's. To this seventy year old, it was an apt rendition to give vent to his feelings of imprisonment. When asked by a bystander where he would go upon 'release', came the instant reply, 'the pub'. He obviously had escaped his daughters that morning to be in the precinct!

Release from lockdown would affect people differently. There was likely to be a phased release affecting various sectors differently. This is how release eventually happened. In the UK by June 2020 we had seen a gradual reduction in number of cases and deaths related to the infection. Therefore progress away from lockdown would be a multi-speed journey with the 'foot on the brake' as it were. The brake would be applied quickly, reversing any release from lockdown, if the rate of infection nationally or locally appeared to be increasing. There was the possibility of differential lockdown in different parts of the UK, depending on local prevalence of infection. Re-imposition of lockdown happened in later months in the UK.

It is said that a general would only go to war if the objectives of the war are clear and there is an effective exit strategy. The purpose of prosecuting a war needs to be quite clear so that consideration can be given to terminate it, when the objectives of the war had been met. The aim of the war may be acquisition of land, a strategic bridge or some other specific objective. Having achieved the objective or not, as the case may be, there would have to be an exit strategy – to extricate oneself from the battle at some point in the future, depending on the circumstances of the time. Failure to achieve the set objectives would be a potent reason to exit from action. We have encountered this in the battle against Covid-19. Take the example of the tracing app that was rolled out by the Department of Health. It just did not achieve its objective, whatever the reasons for this were. But, it was time to withdraw and consider an alternative way of tracing contacts of Convid-19. In war the purpose of an exit strategy is to save life and material; what the military would call "blood and treasure". In the case of the app, new thinking was needed on how the objective of contact tracing could be achieved.

We are engaged in a war – a biological war. The enemy army in this case is the coronavirus. It is silent, invisible and capable of wide spread suffering and death with little respect for international boundaries. The lives of all are at risk. The people on the front line in the battle - medical staff, ambulance, police, fire services etc are the material or 'treasure' that the government seeks to protect and preserve.

The possibility of defeating the virus is remote. The only virus that has been eradicated is small pox. This has been achieved by a successful global immunisation program against the smallpox virus. Similarly other common childhood infectious diseases like German measles (Rubella), measles and polio are contained by effective vaccination programmes in childhood. If any of these infections were to emerge again, it can be concluded that immunisation has not been effective. Such is the power of immunisation to increase herd immunity and virtually eliminate infection while allowing us to safely exist with the viruses. Despite the claims of the anti-vaccination lobby, there is no alternative. There is an increasing and vociferous group of persons who deny the benefits of vaccination and immunisation. At no time in history of the world has there been effective eradication of disease to the extent that vaccination has. Poliomyelitis (polio) is a good example of what can be achieved by vaccination. In June 2020 Nigeria which had polio was declared as being free of wild polio and soon afterwards the whole of Africa was declared free of wild polio virus. Dr.Tedros called it 'a great day... but not the end of polio,' because there continued outbreaks of the infection in West Arica, Afghanistan and Pakistan. To the anti-vaccination group one must pose the question 'how else could these results have been achieved?'

When considering any release from lockdown the government had to walk a tight rope. There needs to be a balance between infection and death and the economy. Get it wrong and either or both would suffer; the eventual effect is increased suffering and deaths. There is a delicate balance between the R number, the number of cases of Covid-19 and the availability of NHS facilities to cover any increase in infections needing hospital and / or intensive care. The economy played an important part in the deliberations. Around the middle of April it was known that many businesses did not have enough available cash to survive more than three months. This was without factoring in supply chain problems which of themselves could put many businesses at risk. Many small businesses like restaurants, hair-dressers, pubs were at risk. Small businesses are the back bone of the economy and it was known that their loss would put any economic recovery at risk. Even for a staged release from lockdown there would need to have been a consistent fall in infections and death rates, an increased ability to test, trace and isolate and reserve NHS capacity. In this challenging environment no one would have wanted to be in the Prime Minister's shoes.

The CMO, Chris Whitty, was explicit when he stated that the UK was going to have to live with the virus. It certainly was not going away and was likely to be circulating until at least the summer of 2021. Therefore he implied that in the short- to medium-term, at least until the spring of 2021, the public would have to be careful. This would mean respecting the new physical distancing of one metre, wearing face masks and so. He also stressed the importance of people reporting when they got symptoms. Reporting of symptoms is vital because of a moral duty to reduce the risk to others.

The difficulties encountered by minsters in trying to plot a gradual way out of lockdown were exposed in the divergence of opinion that was apparent in July 2020.The Prime Minister was keen to get the country back to work with an 'aspirational' time table aiming towards a return to normal life in nine months. However the Chief Scientific Adviser held firm in saying that he thought there was 'absolutely no reason' to stop working from home. He felt that working from home did not affect the productivity of many companies. Although it appeared that the Prime Minister decided to set aside the scientific advice, this was conditional on the 'virus continuing to recede'.

A look at how other countries were proposing to manage any form of exit from lockdown shows how difficult it was going to be sorting out this dilemma. France wanted to open schools on 11th May. Parents and the teaching unions were opposed to the idea of opening schools. Spain proposed to keep schools closed. In Italy schools were not expected to open until September. Sweden had not closed schools at all as it had pursued an alternative way to managing the virus by not having any real lockdown. Sweden depended on the sensibility of its people to look after themselves. Austria allowed small business to start up in Mid April. Germany followed the Austrians.

It is never easy to know when the objective of containing the virus is likely to be achieved. Defeating it comprehensively is unlikely to be a possibility unless there is an effective vaccine. Although the pharmaceutical company, Astra Zeneca had claimed that Britain could be the first country to provide an effective vaccination against Covid-19, this was not likely to be in the short term. Russia claimed it had an effective vaccine around the middle of August 2020. There was much scepticism about this success, especially as trials on safety in humans had not apparently been completed. The world has overcome polio and small pox for example, by mass vaccination of populations. The objective in the battle against Covid-19 is to reduce its infectivity – getting the R number to well below 1. Knowing whether this point has been reached is not easy .No health service in the world is likely to completely eliminate the virus. Does it mean that the country stays in permanent lockdown until the R is negligible? How do we know that, if this hypothetical point is reached, the virus would not shoot another spike? Terminating a military battle is always a political decision. Similarly one can now appreciate the difficulties that politicians face in trying to release from lockdown.

At best, the timing of easing of restrictions and cessation of lockdown is a calculated guess with help from scientific advisors. Scientists cannot give a definite answer to release lockdown regulations or to continue with them. Scientists work only with probabilities and confidence in the predictions they make could be wide and variable. Additionally, of course, the results of scientific modelling can have as many interpretations as there are scientists!

Medical investigators and statisticians are familiar with the term' equipoise'. The term was first used in 1987 by Benjamin Freedman in his paper titled 'Equipoise and the ethics of medical research' which was published in the New England Journal of Medicine. Equipoise is a state of uncertainty as to whether a particular treatment is beneficial or not. It particularly relates to medical trials of efficacy and safety of medicines. The UK was near a state of equipoise towards the end of May 2020. There was a reduction in hospital admissions with signs of reduction in deaths from Covid-19. There was increasing discussion in scientific and political circles about a pathway to easing lockdown. The UK could have continued with comprehensive lockdown as it had been in since 23rd March. Or it could entertain a phased release from it. If the lookdown was continued, one may reach a point where there are no more deaths from the disease and no admissions to hospital with it. But would this be anything more than superficial reassurance? Remember, we know that the virus is still in the community and probably changing or mutating. It can reappear at any time. Or it may be re-introduced into the community. We saw the re-introduction of Covid-19 into New Zealand after many days of being free of the infection. We also learnt about the appearance of Covid-19 in Beijing in June 2020. It is plausible to accept that one may never reach the point of no infection in the UK or for that matter anywhere else. But if lockdown continued, the medical and economic costs would escalate so much that they would combine to pose an even greater threat to the country. Other causes of death would rise due to people not seeking medical help for non-Covid medical conditions like cancer and heart disease. Also the longer the economy is not back to normal the long term effects on health and survival are likely to be grave. In other words Covid-19 could continue to affect our health and survival even after it has diminished in intensity and is not of itself causing illness and death. It could be said that at the end of

May 2020 the UK was at the point of equipoise as regards the battle with Covid-19 was concerned.

In his book 'On War', Carl von Clausewitz talks about the 'Dynamic Law of War'. He describes a state of equilibrium accompanied by a state of tension. In the end of May 2020 there was some 'fluid' equilibrium where there were continued efforts being made to bear down on the virus. The country continued with its precautions like social distancing while scientists continued with research for new armaments in the form of medicines and for a vaccine against the virus. The state of tension continued. There was the possibility that a second spike in infection could arise at any time. Therefore any release from lockdown had to go with a readiness to re-introduce it or to bring in hasher methods of lockdown if the need arose.

In the battle against Covid-19 there is no single, very effective 'magic bullet'. There are no effective antibiotics or anti-viral drugs that could kill the virus. Much was written about the anti-rheumatic drug, hydroxychloroquine. However this drug was proven not to be effective against the virus but at the same time carried serious side effects for e.g. on the heart.

An antiviral drug called remdesivir was found to be capable of preventing multiplication of the virus inside cells in the human body. In the UK, the National Institute of Health and Care Excellence (NICE) recommended its use for treating hospitalised patients with COVID-19. However, NICE advised that further research needed to be done to help understand how effective the drug is in combating Covid-19.

The steroid drug, dexamethasone, was found to be effective in a small group of patients with Covid-19.

Whatever shape release from lockdown took it was never going to be a single event. It was going to be a journey. The destination could also never be the past, pre-Covid state of affairs. Rather there would be a future where we accepted a situation which was described by Dr.Tedros, 'a new normal where we are safer and better prepared'. There would never come a time when any nation could say it is absolutely safe and therefore could return to what was before. The new normal would involve the existing physical measures of distancing, face coverings and scrupulous hygiene and hand washing. The moral duty of everyone to report symptoms and permit follow up of contacts with appropriate isolation would help make everyone safer. Immunisation would greatly help but it would probably have to be a regular feature. And finally health authorities would need to be on the constant lookout for any new viruses and act speedily to contain any chance of spread.

It was therefore important that as the UK approached a managed release from lockdown, the population continued with the social distancing measures that were already in place and to use regular hand washing to reduce contamination with the virus. Face coverings of any suitable description that prevented transmission of the virus to others was recommended and became mandatory in public places in early June 2020. Therefore any release involved continuation of existing personal measures to bear down on the virus and on its spread. The role of every citizen was as important during release from lockdown as it was during it.

If restrictions are lifted too early and there is no regular monitoring of new cases and of deaths, it was possible to envisage a scenario when a second and subsequent waves of Covid-19 appear. In the absence of testing and contact tracing it is almost certain that second and subsequent waves of Covid-19 would occur. During the Spanish flu of 1918 wearing face marks was compulsory in California. This lead to a reduction in the death rate and on 21st November 1918 there were celebrations as people could now do away with their masks. Wearing masks was described as 'four weeks of muzzled misery'. Unfortunately, the flu returned in January 1919 and the death rate in California doubled. It is said in California that the dead of 1919 whisper: "Make sure you don't give up the fight too soon." At the time, Mayor James Rolph claimed that outsiders brought the flu back to San Francisco. He failed to appreciate the major error in easing restrictions too soon.

The UK witnessed re-introduction of lockdown in Leicester in England at the end of June 2020. July 4th was the date when the rest of the UK enjoyed a further liberation from the restrictions of lockdown. The reasons for the re-imposition of lockdown in Leicester were, among others, an increase in the number of cases of the virus; three times the rate as the rest of the country. The problem in Leicester brings into focus the importance of testing, tracing and isolating those who have the virus. This is now accepted as the only way that one could identify pockets of high prevalence of the virus and to bring them under control. Vo in north Italy is a good example of this process. It was a town that was very early on in the pandemic, placed in quarantine. Researchers from the University of Padua and from Imperial College in London tested many people. They found that there were people who carried the virus but did not develop symptoms – asymptomatic people. Then there were those who had the virus and eventually got symptoms of the infection – pre-symptomatic people. Both these groups of persons were potentially able to spread the infection in Vo. But by identifying those who carried the virus and isolating them, the authorities in Vo were able to clamp down on transmission of the virus. Knowing that the virus is likely to reside in the community for many years and in the absence of a vaccine, any form of societal normality can only come from widespread testing, tracing and isolation. In the absence of such a screening process the UK would continue to be on a knife edge.

Long-term protection of public is the number one concern of public health authorities and government. Protection from infections like measles, mumps, diphtheria, polio etc has only been achieved by successful vaccination. It therefore follows that ultimate protection form Covid-19 could only occur with a vaccine, similar to the annual flu vaccination program that we have in the UK. Unlike say polio or measles vaccination the annual flu vaccination does not provide life-long protection or even immunity for longer than a year at most. That is why there is an annual vaccination program so that protection against the virus may be maintained throughout life, especially in those who have underlying medical conditions and are considered vulnerable. Public Health England (PHE) estimated that on average 17,000 people died each year from the flu in England between 2014/15 and 2018/19. Of course, this average figure is from a wide range of 28,330 deaths in 2014/2015 to 1,692 deaths in 208/2019. The seasonal flu has a low mortality rate of about 0.13%. Coronavirus on the other had an initial mortality rate of about 5% when it first appeared in Wuhan. Even with measles, mumps and rubella there are booster vaccinations to enhance protection and ensure that this protection lasts for long periods. What we do not know at present is whether there is effective immunity after Covid-19 and the duration for which this immunity would last. Initial Chinese research suggests that in mild cases of Covid-19 there were no detectable antibodies to the virus. This implies that re-infection could occur as had been reported from South Korea.

South Korea, however, had a very effective contact tracing app which was used successfully to track down cases of Covid-19. It has a population of just over three-quarters of the population in the UK. At the time of this writing South Korea had about 12,500 cases and 280 deaths from Covid-19. It was able to contain the virus by testing up to 100,000 people a day. They coupled this work with contact tracing and were very successful in containing the pandemic. The Deputy Chief Scientific Adviser, Professor Dame Angela McLean said 'I think they are a fine example to us and we should try to emulate what they have achieved.' However the system used in South Korea depended on them having a good public health system. Unfortunately in the UK, this speciality has taken a back seat in recent years and is simply not able to cope with the needs of effective contact tracing at present. Also the South Korean success depended on the authorities having access to CCTV information and information collected from mobile telephones. Some aspects of South Korea's tracing system would be considered significant breaches of data protection regulations and may not be acceptable in the UK.

Contact tracing has previously been tried and found to be useful for e.g. in sexual health clinics and before that in the battle against tuberculosis (TB). Again unfortunately this service has been downgraded. The importance of effective public health devolved locally is now clear. Such a service with local knowledge would have been able to deal with track, trace and isolate more effectively than the centralised system that was introduced in the UK.

Germany commenced a gradual release form lockdown on 27 April when the R number had moved to 0.7. The policy varied between states in the Federation, each of which could decide how they independently implemented advice about release. Shops and schools gradually opened guided by the advice given at the time. On 11th May the Robert Koch Institute (RKI) for disease control reported that R had risen to 1.1. Due to statistical difficulties associated with the R number, RKI was uncertain if the rise in the R value represented a true increase in infections. But caution was advised and the opening of restaurants in Coesfeld, where the R figure rose, was postponed. Germany has an emergency brake which would be deployed if more than 50 infections per 100,000 population per week occur in an area.

In the middle of May 2020 Italy gradually eased its strict lockdown rules. Workers could return to manufacturing and construction jobs, parks and gardens opened and people could visit relatives in the same region. Shop, restaurants, bars etc were allowed to open. It was worrying to read that Italy may have under-reported its number of cases of Covid-19 and its death tally from the infection. A study by the Institute of Public Health and Charite-Universitatsmedizin Berlin said the under-estimates were probably due to a shortage of testing kits or that people died from other causes connected with the pandemic.

By the middle of May, China had not reported any new cases for a month. Schools had re-opened allowing students to sit their examinations. Domestic flights had returned to 60% of pre-Covid-19 levels although passenger numbers were not available. However, much scepticism has been expressed about the figures coming out of China, which may not have been representative of the true scale of the pandemic there and of the real numbers of patients that had died as a result of it.

On 27th April New Zealand Prime Minister, Jacinda Arden, said that the country had avoided the worst effects of the pandemic as she prepared to ease restrictions the same day. The country moved from the Level 4 alert status down to Level 3, as she asked all to be vigilant due to risks from people being in contact with others. In Level 3 some retailers and restaurants together with schools were allowed to open, on a small scale.

Denmark was one of the earliest countries in Europe to commence its journey out of lockdown. It planned to open primary schools on 15th April. The Danish Prime Minister Ms Mette Frederiksen was of the view that having acted early to contain the crisis, the country was in a position to progress towards release. She acknowledged that it would be gradual with physical distancing and testing continuing so as to keep the R number down

Professor David Robertson, head of viral genomics and bioinformatics at the University of Glasgow, told the House of Lords that 'Covid-19 could be around for years to come'. He compared it with Ebola which causes symptoms and is readily identified. Covid-19, on the other hand, may not cause symptoms and so is difficult to identify.

He added: "If you contrast with Ebola, which has very high virulence, kills many, many people, it makes it very controllable and you can very readily identify the infected people. He said 'I think we have to be clear that we're not going to be able to eradicate this virus. It's going to settle into the human population and in several years it will become a normal virus.' This means that the world is never going to be free of the corona virus. The UK's Deputy Chief Medical Office, Professor Jonathan Van-Tam said that the UK must be prepared for a second wave of the virus infection in autumn and/ or winter of 2020 like the seasonal flu virus. He expressed the view that people have got to get accustomed to living with the virus in their midst.

Information about the nature of the virus is rapidly changing and in the months that follow the world was likely to better understand its nature. We would then be able to understand how it induces immunity in people who are infected with it. We would also be likely to know how effective immunity would be and how much protection would be provided against getting the infection again. Until such time the most effective protective measures are those designed to reduce transmission of the virus.

In this uncertain climate governments across the world had to deal with release from lockdown.

The Prime Minister, Boris Johnson, introduced the first changes to lockdown rules on the 28th of May 2020.

With the UK government planning an easing of restrictions from the 1st of June, the Deputy Chief Medical Officer, Professor Jonathan Van-Tam said that the country was facing a 'very dangerous moment'. He was mindful of the difficult decision confronting the UK government as it must have been for governments around the world as they individually grappled with how to commence release from lockdown. With about 50 scientists in SAGE, each having their own interpretation of the available data and of the balance of risk and benefit from easing restrictions, it must have been extremely difficult for the Cabinet to have made the decision to begin release from lockdown on 1st June. Professor Van-Tam expressed the responsibilities of all those involved in what was an experiment in release. The government needed to be cautious in its actions, scientists need to monitor the situation very closely and the public had to act responsibly in following the guidance provided. In colourful language, Prof. Van-Tam pleaded with the public 'Don't tear the pants out of it, and don't go further than the guidance actually says.'

At this stage, in the absence of testing and contact tracing, it was a gamble to know if easing of lockdown restrictions would cause a rise in infections. Sir Jeremy Farrar said that there was a need to have a tracing system in place prior to easing lockdown. He felt that the infection was still spreading too fast In England, to begin to ease lockdown.

The government in Wales described a stepwise traffic light process for managing movement out of lockdown. There would be a gradual progression from red to amber and finally to green if there were no crises of infection during the journey of release. The unlocking 'roadmap' as it was called was described as a 'cautious, coherent approach' which puts 'the health of the public first'. Mark Drakeford, the First Minister of Wales, implied that 'normal life will not be possible for many months – possibly years.' This statement acknowledges that the state of equipoise in dealing with Covid-19 may continue for a long time yet and that there is not likely to be anything like normal life for many years. Indeed the experience of Covid-19 may have altered people's impressions and attitudes to the extent that a kind of natural 'self censorship' of behaviour would occur. For e.g. the use of face coverings, maintaining some physical distance from others and regular hand washing are likely to become a regular feature of life. This is a good change which would help for e.g. in reducing transmission of other infections too. In the case of sepsis for example, hand washing is known to be crucial in stemming transmission of bacteria.

Scotland approached release from lockdown much slowly. It started with allowing people to exercise more than once a day from the middle of May. The First Minister of Scotland, Nicola Sturgeon, advised public in May to continue to stay at home unless it was really necessary to go out e.g. for food or medicines. This decision was based on the fact the R number was still not sufficiently low to allow the government in Scotland to begin easing restrictions further.

In Northern Ireland the regulations remained unchanged in May.

Although there were minor differences in the lockdown regulations, in the four nations of the UK there appeared to be a desire to reassure the public that easing would follow when the infection rate as judged by the R number was sufficiently low to ensure safety in doing so. The imperative of the moment was to try and avoid a resurgence of infection. Secondly there was the feeling that 'lockdown fatigue' may be setting in, with not infrequent breaches of the regulations taking place. Hence there was a need to set out a road map of release from lockdown.

In addition to a falling R number all were agreed that there needed to be a reduction in hospital admissions for Covid-19, for at least a fortnight. There was also a need to have a sufficient reserve capacity in hospital to manage any unexpected surge in infections. And finally there was the need to have a reasonable stockpile of PPE etc to help deal with any increase in hospital in-patient activity as a result of the infection.

Another vital factor that most likely to have been considered was the availability of front-line staff to manage any surge that may occur. Staff had been working almost at breakneck speed from the onset of the pandemic. They were likely to have been mentally and physically exhausted. A break from front line duties was urgently needed by these personnel. Any sudden spike in infection would have placed an unbearable strain on already exhausted staff.

At the end of the day, after all consideration, the decision to move away from lockdown and the manner in which it is done could only be a political one. Come out of lockdown too early and a second or third wave of Covid-19 might emerge. In the Spanish flu of 1918 the third wave claimed many deaths including the deaths of many young persons. Delay release from lockdown and the financial and economic price could be so great as to keep the country in indebtedness for a long time. This would mean reduction in services especially on health and social care, which would have had adverse effects on the population. Also during lockdown other chronic diseases like cancer, heart disease do not get the timely attention than would otherwise have been the case. This would in turn work through as worsening illness and an increased drain on the NHS, when its resources would have been stretched. Investment in the NHS would be limited unless financed by even more borrowing. Financial markets would exact a heavy price for this, which would have to be paid by future generations. The young generation may complain about lockdown and that their way of life and their opportunities are stymied. But would they accept recurring waves of infection and a continuing threat to life?

Additionally would they accept the financial costs of spikes of recurrent infection like higher rates of interest and of income tax?

Even a phased and gradual release from lockdown is not an easy decision to make. But it is one that had to be made. It would require a conversation with the public on the risks and benefits of being in lockdown as opposed to coming off it. Scientific information may help but what the future hold is uncertain. Those who clamour for a hasty release from lockdown need to be aware of the sword of Damocles hanging over the head of the government. Get it wrong and the government would be held responsible for a recurrence of the pandemic and all that follows from this.

An initial plan was suggested by the Chancellor of the Exchequer, Rishi Sunak, which involved maintaining the social distance of 2 metres even in the workplace. Businesses that deal with the public could open within existing limitations. Therefore other shops and even fast food chains may open without risk to the public or to those who work in them. The government's scientific advisors stated that a reduction of the separating distance between individuals from two metres to one metre would significantly increase the chance of becoming infected from another person. But the WHO recommends a separating distance of one metre. In Belgium, Germany, Greece and the Netherlands restaurants are permitted to open with a 1.5 metre physical distancing rule. In Austria, Denmark, France, Hong Kong and Singapore the separating distance is one metre. With no social distancing in place the chances of catching infection from another infected person is 13%. This figure reduces to 2.6% when there is a separation of 1 metre and 1.3% with a 2 metres separation. The risk of becoming infected drops markedly to less than 1% with a three metre separation and becomes negligible with further increase in the separating distance between two individuals. The risk of catching the infection when wearing a mask is 3% when compared to a 17% risk if no mask is worn.

A study published in the medical Journal, Lancet, showed that keeping a distance of greater than one metre from another person was associated with a lower risk of catching the infection than when the separation distance was one metre. Commenting on the Lancet study Professor Trish Greenhalgh and colleagues from the University of Oxford said that staying one metre apart from other people reduced the chances of catching Covid-19 to 80%. Wearing a face mask or other face covering reduces the risk of catching the infection by up to 85%. Professor Linda Bauld from the University of Edinburgh stressed the importance of physical distancing and urged that the current separation of 2 metres be maintained wherever possible. However, Professors Carl Heneghan and Tom Jefferson from the Centre for Evidence Based Medicine at Oxford University state that most of the evidence on physical distancing is outdated and not related to Covid-19. They say that keeping 1 metre apart can reduce the risk of catching Covid-19 by 80%. The chance of contracting the virus is 1.3% when 2 metre away from an infected person. This risk increased to only 2.6% when the separating distance was reduced to 1 metre. Dr Mike Lonergan, a statistician and epidemiologist from the University of Dundee in Scotland also was doubtful about the evidence on separating distance. He concluded that avoiding physical contact with others is important to prevent infection and a one metre separation between individuals is better than simply avoiding contact. There was no evidence to support the assertion that two metres apart was better than one metre in preventing transmission of infection. Dr. Lonergan stated that 78 per cent of the reduction in risk of infection happens below one metre. If the distance between individuals was increased there was only an 11% chance of reduction in transmission of the virus.

Where did 2 metre rule originate from? In the 1940's a bacteria, not a virus, called haemolytic streptococcus was common and causes tonsillitis, rheumatic heart disease and kidney disease, among others. Rheumatic heart disease causes permanent heart valve damage. The disease is still prevalent in some parts of the world. In 1948, when investigating the spread of the germ, it was found that many people produced large droplets, most of which did not travel further than five and a half feet or 1.7 metres. But in a small minority of participants the germ was found almost 10 feet away or 3 metres. This led to a safe 2 metre cut off which is the basis of advice against Covid-19 spread today. However science has moved a long way since 1948 and we are better able to understand droplet movements. Spread of droplets is affected by the rate of expulsion from the nose and mouth, humidity, air flow in the room etc. So a cough or a sneeze would propel infected droplets from a person with Covid-19 a greater distance than it would during normal silent breathing. Also, air that is breathed out has droplets of varying size which will progress over varying distances affected not only by the force of propulsion but also by gravity.

The evidence to support rigid advice on physical distancing is limited.

This was undoubtedly a confusing area, a veritable minefield of statistics and with claims and counter claims. All this information was as confusing to the scientists themselves as it must have been to those who received it, the Cabinet which had to make a decision. There were no right or wrong answers to this dilemma. What would the average person have made of all of this information, or more interestingly, what would the man on the Clapham omnibus have made of it? Who is this man on the Clapham omnibus? 'The Clapham omnibus has many passengers. The most venerable is the reasonable man, who was born during the reign of Victoria but remains in vigorous health. Amongst the other passengers are the right-thinking member of society, familiar from the law of defamation, the officious bystander, the reasonable parent, the reasonable landlord, and the fair-minded and informed observer, all of whom have had season tickets for many years.' The man is a fictional character but is useful as a person who is reasonable and in the context of Covid-19 would have wanted to act in a safe manner. What we know of Covid-19 and what is an incontrovertible fact is that close contact with others increases the risk of catching the infection if that other is either infected, with or without symptoms. It is also known that virus generating activities, also called aerosol generating procedures or AGP like coughing, sneezing or even conversing in close proximity without protection exposes one to the virus. Finally, touching objects and touching the face, nose or eyes carries the risk of transmitting the virus from those objects to one's face from whence it may be inspired into the lungs. Therefore a reasonable person, the man on the Clapham omnibus, would keep some separation between himself and others outside his bubble. And his bubble would have been those he shared his home with and who were free of infection. He would wash his hands frequently and use face covering when out and about.

Irrespective of the practice in other countries there is no doubt that physical distancing of people is one of the important factors in curtailing the spread of infection. Social distancing with use of masks and regular hand washing would become essential activities in daily life to help diminish the risk of spread of Covid-19. These health practices would become an integral part of the 'new normal'. The government has to decide what level of distancing it is prepared to accept to encourage business to function and to kick-start the economy. It is obvious that a social distance greater than two metres, while appearing to provide maximum protection against the risk of infection, is not acceptable. The adverse impact on the economy would be too great. On the other hand reducing the physical distance below one metre carries a great risk of the transmission of infection between persons. But a reduced distance would allow many businesses, especially the hospitality industry to return to near normal levels of activity. The government has to choose between the Scylla of an increased risk of Covid-19 in the population and the Charybdis of a severely depressed economy. This was especially relevant in the latter half of June 2020 when the WHO warned that the world was at a dangerous time in the pandemic as the virus was spreading worldwide and many people were susceptible to infection. The economy was near-stagnant and could have been entering a 'dangerous time'. At the time of this writing more than 8.5 million people around the world had been infected and nearly half a million had died. Around the same time we heard that Beijing's confidence in overcoming the pandemic was shattered by the news that there was a new outbreak of Covid-19. On 19th June there were a total of 183 cases of the infection. The public in Beijing were assured by the leading epidemiologist, Wu Zunyou, that the number of new case would soon diminish. This was not to be the case as on 18th June there were 21 cases while on 19th June there were 25 new cases. This showed how easily recurrence of infection can occur and that stringent preventive measures need to be maintained for the foreseeable future.

It is in this febrile and worrying environment that the government had to navigate through a careful path out of lockdown.

Would the UK or indeed the world be able to return to pre-Covid days? Release from lockdown is not likely to be an event but a process which could last for some years. The duration of the 'process of release' from lockdown, is likely to be determined by the R number, the reproduction rate of the virus. This in turn would be influenced by how well public complies with advice on prevention of spread. The duration of release from lockdown would be considerably shortened if and when a successful vaccine is discovered and it is shown to induce enduring immunity in those who have it. Dr.Tedros talked about the need for 'national unity' and 'global solidarity' if the world is to 'finish this pandemic in less than two years'. Yet again the world is reminded that we are all in this altogether.

In the UK we are witnessing several local outbreaks, especially in the north-west of the country, in Greater Manchester and Lancashire. We saw it in Leicester. Internationally there are recurrences of varying magnitude in Spain and New Zealand for example. These spikes in infection may be minor episodes but could spread to give a significant second national spike of the pandemic- what is called a 'U' spike. In the Spanish flu of 1918 there were three spikes – a 'W' pattern of recurrences of infection. Could we have the same with Covid-19 or could we have multiple 'W' spikes? While waiting for a successful vaccine and for newer treatments for the complications of Covid-19, the only available tools in the armamentarium are the keeping a physical distance from others, wearing face coverings and hand washing. These aspects of prevention are not to be considered lightly; they are the only ones that are available to each and everyone in society. Applied together they can be very effective in curbing the spread of and eventually the mortality form Covid-19. They would also help to resuscitate the economy.

The rise in infections is the real risk as the UK or indeed any country moves to ease lockdown restrictions. As always exit from lockdown must be associated with individual persistence with the physical measures to limit the spread of infection. In the early days of the pandemic the reproduction rate of the virus or the R figure was between 3 and 4. With lockdown measures in place the figure had dropped to between 0.7 and 1 in May. However around the middle of August the figure in the UK was between 0.9 and 1. With autumn imminent and the seasonal flu time approaching, having an R figure at or above 1 was worrying. While there have been local lockdowns in Leicester, Manchester, and Oldham etc one needs to be worried that any significant surge would inevitably lead to another national lockdown, with all its attendant consequences which all of us would be keen to avoid. It was felt that young persons, who erroneously consider themselves immune from the infection, are responsible for the R level being stubbornly high. Dr.Hans Kluge, WHO Regional Director for Europe, said that he was very concerned that under-24s are now appearing as new cases of the infection. He stressed that although the virus may be a low risk to the young it did not mean that there is no risk as the virus 'may stick to your body like a tornado with a long tail'. The two additional risks are first, it is not known whether a mild form that youngsters get may still not leave them with serious consequences. Secondly of course is the greater risk that the young people may be spilling the virus to elderly parents and grandparents at home and to the community at large. It is worth recalling the words of Rebecca Solnit who wrote that in a disaster there is a 'minority whose callousness and self-interest often become a second disaster."

One of the first tentative steps in the move away from lockdown was the opening of schools. This sparked much debate with the teaching unions rightly claiming that their members, the teachers, would be exposed to undue risk by returning to school. It is known that children have some degree of inherent resistance to the virus. The number of children who have suffered with Covid-19 is extremely low. But children could be spreaders of infection and hence the concern of teachers unions. Children can have the same amount of viral load in them as adults but tend to suffer fewer infections. Also, research points towards children being less likely to spread the infection. For e.g. a study from the University of Queensland, which had yet to be peer reviewed, found that children were the source of infection in less than 10% of cases. But, the WHO had cautioned against assuming that children cannot transmit Covid 19.

Professor Russell Viner, from the University College London, Great Ormond Street Institute of Child Health, said that their research 'shows children and young people appear 56 per cent less likely to contract Covid-19 from infected others'. Children are less likely to transmit the virus and less likely to contribute to proliferating the pandemic, although there is much that is uncertain, he wrote.

Parents had varying views on return to school. About 25% of parents have difficulty in encouraging and supporting their children to learn at home. A similar percentage of parents say that they are not equipped for the role of supporting education of their children while at home. Many parents are naturally concerned about too early a release from lockdown but are also worried about their children's education and how much they may be missing by not attending school. Many parents do not want their children to attend school until September 2020.

SAGE has warned about the harmful effects of continuing lockdown on children's education and the effect this would have for their further education and therefore for their employments prospects in later life.

Professor of Public Health, Robert Dingwall, said children are more likely to die from lightning strikes than from the coronavirus in schools.

Smaller children would not be compelled to wear face masks when schools commence, although decisions would be left to the discretion of individual head teachers.

The UK government proposed that as from the 1st June 2020 early providers open for children of all ages. Primary schools were encouraged to open during the key transition years of nursery, and years 1 and 6.

From 15th June classes for pupils in years 10 and 12 would return to school

Return to school would need compliance with social distancing rules. However education authorities acknowledge that this would be difficult for little children and those of primary school age. It would be left to head teachers to decide how many children would be allowed to attend each day.

Children or adults with symptom suggestive of Covid-19 and those who have someone at home with features of Covid-19 should not attend school.

Government suggested that class sizes should not exceed 15 pupils to allow for social distancing.

However many local authorities in the north west of England had advised in the first week of June, schools not to open because the virus was still present in these areas and the R figure was still around 1.

Scotland, on the other hand had planned for all its children to return to school in August. In Wales all schools were set to open on 29th June. However, the PM warned that this could be delayed if there was a second and subsequent waves in the infection. The PM spoke after people were found crowding the beaches in the last week of June with no adherence to physical separation. Brawls occurred and some people were stabbed. This entailed responses from the emergency services, which in turn placed those personnel at un-called for risk. Also PHE had reported an increase in coronavirus infections in schools since they opened on the 1st of June.

It was hoped that all schools could re-open in September 2020. However, it was recognised in June that even this would be at risk if there was a spike in infections caused by failure of the public to maintain a reasonable physical distance from others. But schools in England opened in the first week of September to much joy in children. Happy to return to their familiar learning environments and to their friends whom they had not met for several months, the smiles on the faces of school children was a sight to behold.

The 'moral duty' of children returning to school, that the PM talked about, had been accomplished.

The Prime Minister said that there was a moral duty of society to send children back to school. That this is incontrovertible is supported by the Leader of the Opposition, Sri Kier Starmer, who said that this should be so without 'if or buts'.

With evidence that children are not at great risk of spreading the infection to others it is useful to focus on physical distancing. What is a safe separating distance to prevent transmission of infection? This can probably be answered by knowing how far the virus could spread from an infected person to another. From the outset the WHO maintained that a 1 metre separating distance was needed to prevent droplet spread from an infected person to another. As Lydia Bourouiba from the Massachusetts Institute of Technology said that the hot, moist air that comes from the lungs when a person breathes out contains a range of droplet sizes from visible ones to invisible mist. These droplets can travel varying distances depending on the speed at which they are released. Air is expelled for e.g. at a much slower speed in normal breathing than when a person sneezes. A person expels about 3000 droplets in a single cough at speeds of up to 50 miles per hour (0.8 km per hour). During a sneeze air speed reaches 100 miles per hour (1.6km per hour). The virus could therefore travel a considerable distance and naturally concerns have been raised that it could even reach a distance of 26 feet. Few would agree that that there is a serious risk of contamination at 26 feet from the index person. Derek Chu writing in The Lancet concluded that 'a physical distance of more than 1 meter (just over 3 feet) probably results in a large reduction in virus infections. For every 3 feet more, the relative effect "might" increase as much as two times'.

What we therefore know is that increasing distance diminishes the risk of infection. But that is not the whole story. As Zeshan Qureshi, Nicholas Jones and others from the Centre for Evidence Based Medicine in

Oxford wrote, other factors like viral load in the infected person, number of persons and extent of crowding, whether indoors or outdoors and the use of face coverings help to reduce the risk.

Partial release from lockdown in UK came on the 1st June 2020. From this date in England, six people were allowed to meet outside so long as they abide with social distancing rules of keeping apart at 2 meters. Some primary schools also opened. Release was a gradual process. But there was opposition even to this measured step. Prof John Edmunds, from the London School of Hygiene & Tropical Medicine, was of the view that as the number of cases of Covid-19 was still high, he thought the decision to release was 'political". There was considerable opposition to the release from lockdown at this stage as the test and trace system was still not bedded in and it was not known at the time if the system was effective. That this was a dangerous time was recognised by scientists as the rate of infection could change either way. There was caution expressed by all that this managed release from lockdown needed to be handled judiciously. It was not to be total freedom for the public and there was not to be a return to how life was before the onset of lockdown.

The number of new cases was 8000 per day at the beginning of release from lockdown. This was with a R figure at 1 or just below it. This was considered by some to be too high to come out of lockdown. Ideally one would have like to have seen no new cases before release. Modelling was done with a death rate from the disease of 1%; this means that 80 people would die. However this does not take into account that as at 1st June the total, mortality rate in the UK was 13%; 39,369 people had died from Covid-19 out of a total of 277,985 who had the disease. This may not have been an accurate figure because testing was still in its infancy and the number of asymptomatic and mildly symptomatic cases was not known. Globally 380,318 had died out of a total of 6,382,951 giving a death rate of 5.95%. Looking at these figures it would appear optimistic and unsafe to release from lockdown, as the UK did. The death rate could rise astronomically leading to say 450-1000 deaths daily from the 8000 new cases. This would be in addition to the deaths in patients who had the infection prior to 1st June.

Eight thousand new cases each day may indicate that the infection is still spreading fast and that release from lockdown was a risk. SAGE had emphasised the need for a good test and trace system to be in place before any consideration was given to release from lockdown. This is the strategy that has been followed in some other countries.

It is now possible to appreciate the resistance of the Chief Medical Officer, Chris Whitty, to any initial lowering of the alert level in the country. Doctors would look at the whole issue from a pandemic and patient safety point of view. A politician, on the other hand, is driven by economic and political considerations. However, the inescapable fact is that more cases equates with more deaths.

But on 3rd June, just two days after the start of release from lockdown, the Chief Scientific Officer, Sir Patrick Vallance warned that the infection rate was not coming down as fast as he would have liked it to be. The R factor was still hovering around 1. Also, testing had shown that more than 1800 people a day had returned positive tests. In this situation it was right for Chris Whitty to insist that the alert level remain unchanged at 4.

Too early a general release from lockdown carries the risk in a spike in infection and with it an increase in deaths. This would necessitate an additional lockdown with all the disruption and cost related to it. Any rise in R above 1 would be a signal to bring back lockdown. Now, return of lockdown does not have to be uniformly applied nationally. It could be applied differently in localities where the infection rate is high. In early June R was between 0.7 and 0.9. But even a range of R between 0.7 and 0.9 provides only limited assurance as these figures are approximations linked to a great level of uncertainty. When the R figure is, say, below 0.5 we can be assured that the UK is in a comfort zone. This too would, however, need regular review. But the average of 0.7-0.9 still concealed areas of the country where R was higher than 1 for e.g. in the northwest and in the south west. The government was caught in between a rock and a hard place in trying to decide the rate of release from lockdown. Continuing lockdown now carried increasingly dire economic consequences. And the financial support scheme provided by government for businesses could not continue for too long; after all furlough was a form of subsidised, state sponsored unemployment that was used for the greater good. It was a short term measure until the general environment of safety from the virus improved.

Modelling by Cambridge University in early June suggested that there were 17,000 new cases of Covid-19 a day. With this rate of infection and limited testing and tracing, any further release from lockdown could be very risky. The rate of infection would have had to be monitored extremely closely. On the other hand, the government would have needed conviction and a strong resolve to re-impose any form of lockdown at short notice. It was reassuring to hear Matt Hancock, the Health Secretary, say that the government was not placing the economy above the health of people.

It is a matter of regret that getting out of lockdown became harder than it could have been because the country did not go into lockdown earlier than it did. Nor did the UK have all the facilities in place to test and trace cases of infection.

There is no doubt that exit from lockdown is important for the economy. The UK went into lockdown with a debt-to-GDP ratio of 86% compared say with Germany's 59%. The debt-to-GDP ratio in UK would rise the longer it stays in lockdown.

The R figure varies across the country. In the West Country it was reported to be hovering around 0.8 -1.1 in early June 2020. In the North East and Yorkshire it varied between 0.7 and 1 while in the East it was between 0.7 and 0.9. The rate for London, the South East, and the Midlands and in the North West was 0.7-1. These figures show that the R figure is still not significantly below 1 at the time of writing. It is not a figure that provides comfort as it could easily go up and increase the number of cases and with it the numbers of deaths from the infection. The ONS stated that between 25th May and 7th June it estimated that 33,000 persons had the virus during the period. This gave an infection rate of 1 in 1700 persons compared to the ONS figure of 1 in 400 persons infected in the middle of May 2020 when it was estimated that 133,000 people were infected. It therefore appeared that the rate of infection was coming down. This had to be a hopeful sign but one would have liked to see the R figure significantly down and staying low before we could have assumed that the UK was likely to be over the worst of the epidemic. This was however no guarantee against a second spike as the virus and the infection continued to reside in the community.

Some areas of England had seen no cases of infection. Rutland had no cases for two weeks while Torbay in Devon had not seen a case of the infection for four weeks to the middle of June. At the same time 60 % of local councils were reporting on average once case of infection a day or even less. This was all good news but had to be taken with caution. There may be cases of the infection even in areas with no reported cases. This is where an effective test and track system would have proven its worth. It is likely that as the weeks go by more areas would report lesser numbers or no cases. Regional variations in lockdown were opposed by the Prime Minister. This was a natural point of view as it was likely to cause frictions between communities. However if there arose marked variations in rates of infections between localities, a strategy would have been required short of a general lockdown for all. A general lockdown would have been difficult to justify in areas that remained free of infection.

However, in areas where there is a recurrence of infection and the risk that Covid-19 may be spreading, the government and the Prime Minister have made clear they would use a targeted lockdown, called a 'whack a mole' strategy. This would involve severe restrictions locally and would include prisons, care homes and whole towns if needed. This approach would help contain and eventually eliminate local outbreaks that could otherwise threaten the whole country.

In the light of the reducing R number and the diminution in the numbers of people infected, SAGE advised that individual companies should be left to decide how they could operate safely. For e.g. a change of physical distancing from 2metres to 1metre would allow car manufacturing companies and factories producing components for cars to move safely from 50 % production to near 100 % production capacity. Bus and train operators could go up to 40 % capacity from the current 10-20% using the 2-metre rule. The one-metre rule is considered safe by the WHO. This however did not mean that the UK should jump hastily to a one –metre rule. In Australia where they had far fewer deaths than in the UK, a physical separation of 1.5 metre was still in place. New Zealand relaxed its distancing rules completely on 8th June. It was one of about eight other countries including Montenegro, Papua New Guinea, the Seychelles and Fiji which had seen no active cases of Covid-19. However, in New Zealand, while physical distancing was suspended, its borders remain closed imposing great difficulty on its tourism industry. Any relaxation of distancing rules is only one small measured step on a journey towards a more widespread release from lockdown.

Release from lockdown had to be managed gradually. There were cases of recurrence of infections after apparent absences of it. In Beijing three new cases were reported on 11th June after fifty-five days without any infections. A rise in cases in Tulsa, Oklahoma in the USA was attributed to indoor events. In the USA, California, Texas and Florida which eased lockdown measures, are seeing a rise in infection rates. Australia had proceeded cautiously by allowing up to 10,000 people into sports stadiums as long as physical distancing is maintained. And we needed to be aware of Sweden and Poland where the peak of the virus had still not passed in the second week of June. Sweden did not have physical distancing rules. New Zealand reported on 16th June that it had two new cases of Covid-19. Both had travelled to the country via Doha in Qatar and Brisbane from the UK, to visit a dying patient. Exception had apparently been made to allow the travellers to enter the country. Extensive tracing and testing of all possible contacts was done. New Zealand did not hesitate to enlist the help of its military to help in tracing possible infection in the country. These two cases ended a consecutive 24-day period when New Zealand did not have any case of the infection. The recurrence of infection in New Zealand showed very clearly that any release from lockdown had to be managed extremely carefully. New Zealand had 102 days free of new infections before it showed a resurgence of Covid-19 mainly in Auckland. In Beijing there was an outbreak of over 30 cases on 15th June and a similar number the next day. These were said to have originated in a large wholesale food market in the city. Testing was started immediately to try and isolate possible cases of the infection and so help stem its spread. Despite having a low number of cases and of deaths, Chancellor Angela Merkel urged Germans to respect social distancing rules and to remain cautious. Following discussion she had with the heads of the various states in Germany, agreement was reached to prevent any large events until the end of October. In Hong Kong the third wave of infection, which is the largest spike in the country, was due to infections spread by ship and air crews. Hong Kong is one of the largest commercial shipping ports in the world. Hong Kong airport is an important hub in Asia. Considering the large numbers of crew movements in these two localities it is easy to see how re introduction of the virus happened.

The possibility of recurrence of infection is considered real by all and must remain a priority in the UK as the numbers of infection appear to be diminishing.

The alternative SAGE committee has Sir David King, the government's previous Chief Scientific Adviser as one of its members. Modelling by this group showed that localised outbreaks were likely to occur. And these would have had to be managed by local councils and away from direct central control. This appeared to be a sensible prediction of likely events and a reasonable means of managing recurrence of infection. Local outbreaks occurred and were managed by local departments of Public Health.

The re-imposition of lockdown regulations in Leicester was a useful study of how lockdown operated there. Leicester is a city with a large immigrant population, form India, Pakistan and Bangladesh. Many have retained their culture and ways of living. For example if temples and mosques were closed during lockdown, this did not prevent people gathering in their living rooms to pray, with scant regard for physical distancing. The other area of particular concern is the many, some would say about one thousand, garment factories in the area. Some of these factories were described as nothing more than sweat shops like those that we have heard about operating in parts of south Asia. Work continued in these factories during lockdown. It was thought most garment factories were operating at their normal capacity by 22nd April. This is although lockdown was imposed on 23rd of March and these establishments should have been closed. The working conditions at these factories were at best described as unhygienic. Workers were cramped with limited physical distancing, if at all and with little or no regard for health and safety. Toilet facilities for workers were sparse and unhygienic. The workers themselves lived in crowded houses where even twenty people lived in a three-bedroom house with a single toilet. The income earned by the garment factory workers was less that the national minimum wage and sometimes as low as £2 per hour. The garment workers campaign group called 'Labour Behind The Label' claimed for e.g. that one fashion group was operating at 80% capacity during lockdown. To describe some of the living and working conditions in the garment factories as amounting to modern slavery would not be out of context. The big, unanswered question is why the authorities did not enforce the regulations to ensure that the people of Leicester were safe. Was this another example of political correctness?

The area that caused much discussion in the UK was the plan to quarantine arrivals into the country for fourteen days. Currently the Foreign and Commonwealth Office advises against all but essential travel abroad. However all passengers, including UK nationals, will have to provide an address where they would have been staying and therefore where they would have had to self- isolate for 14 days after arrival in the UK. A specific form was to be provided for this information and any passenger refusing to provide information or to fill the form would have been fined £1000. Spot checks would be made to the addresses provided and any person who is not found to be self- isolating would have been fined £1000. Self- isolation in this context meant not going to work, to any public areas, not using public transport etc. Sick pay would not be provided for this period. The only persons exempt from the need to quarantine were those passengers who arrived in the UK from the Common Travel Area (CTA) so long they had been previously been resident in the CTA for fourteen days immediately prior to travel to the UK. The CTA comprises the Republic of Ireland, the Channel Islands and the Isle of Man.

The government was also trying to make special arrangements with other countries with low infection rates. These so called 'air bridges' would allow travel from those countries without having to quarantine upon return to the UK.

Some persons were exempt from the quarantine regulation. These were medical personnel, haulage and freight workers, seasonal workers etc. These are persons who are essential for the delivery of health care and for the economy. These persons are not by any means all free of the virus. Testing should have been available so that those exempt from quarantine could be deemed to be safe from the risk of spreading the virus. The third wave in Hong Kong is evidence that no group of persons are safe from the risk of spreading. The only way to ensure a person is not at risk to others is to have tested negative for the virus. Additionally, of course, the availability of serial testing would ensure that a person remains safe.

For too long society has become accustomed to taking no risks. If something went wrong, then someone had to be called to account. Progress would be slow in an extreme risk- averse society. If the phrase 'nothing ventured, nothing gained' is to mean something in this crisis, it is that, as Theodore Roosevelt said 'there comes a time in the life of a nation, as in the life of an individual, when it must face great responsibilities'. Our forefathers did not progress without taking risks. This is a time when a calculated risk has to be taken. On the information that was available it is possible that the virus would never have been eliminated and that we would have had to get used to living with it. To wait for negligible infection would have been folly; to wait for zero infection would have been madness. Waiting would have nearly decimated the economy and with it the standard of living leading to worsening public health. 'Decision is often the difference between greatness and mediocrity'. This was the time to act on lockdown.

On 23rd June the UK government set out the details of the next steps of its release from lockdown on 4th July. The Prime Minister said that he wanted Britons to get out and to 'enjoy themselves' and for 'bustle and activities' to return to towns and cities. Hotels, bars, restaurants would open with certain conditions. Hairdressers, cinemas and theme parks would open from 4th July which was dubbed 'Super Saturday'. The two metre physical distancing was reduced to just one metre. All this happened while the Chief Medical Officer, Chris Whitty, again warned that the country should expect to be dealing with Covid-19 and to be at risk for a long time. He meant that the country would not be into a safer zone until well in to 2021.

The knife edge on which the country was at the end of June was worrying. Especially as we saw half a million people were on the Dorset coast on 25th June enjoying the sunshine. This was a recipe for disaster which prompted the Health Secretary to warn of possible re-imposition of lockdown. The effects of this would have been to delay opening of schools, risk to jobs, higher unemployment etc.

Coincidentally the next day the DG of the WHO, Dr.Tedros, said that the WHO expected to see one million new cases worldwide in the next week with the total number of cases in the world exceeding 10 million. He said that in the first month of the pandemic there were 10,000 cases worldwide while now there were 4 million cases in the past month. The figures he said was a 'sober reminder' that Covid-19 were still around. He emphasised yet again the need for testing and tracing to overcome the crisis.

Sweden remains an interesting experiment in the handling of the pandemic. It does not have to go through the burdens of release from lockdown as it did not impose national lockdown. How did it manage and how would it fare in the long term were recurring questions. It is close to its Scandinavian neighbours but different to them in how the pandemic was handled. So also Germany and Belgium are close to each other physically as countries but had different infection rates as were Spain and Portugal.

Each country has to manage exit from lockdown differently depending on local circumstances, infection rates and compliance by the public.

o0:0o

DEATH AND DEBT

A mathematics teacher asked his pupils in secondary school to imagine numerical infinity. What is the figure of infinity? Could it be written on a paper? No, for it would take all the paper in the world and more to write the numerical value of infinity, if it was ever possible to do so.

Now imagine the lesser figure of a trillion. What is it? One knows a million, probably knows a billion, but what is a trillion? If there are six zeros in a million, how many are there in a trillion? A million is 1,000,000. A trillion is 1,000,000,000,000. That is one followed by 12 zeros. The digit 1 followed by 100 zeros would be a googol. This is not the largest number, which is a googolplex which is the digit one followed by a googol of zeros. The term googolplex was coined by Milton Sirotta, the nephew of the American mathematician Edward Kasner. There is currently no use for a googolplex as it is so large. It is in fact probably larger that the total number of atoms in the universe.

Could the 'Man who knew Infinity', Srinivasa Ramanujam, have comprehended what a trillion is?

Coming down to earth and the UK specifically, the national debt was in excess of £ 2 trillion in the middle of August 2020. This is almost as if each household in the UK was in debt to the tune of £72,000. This level of debt came about from the generous support schemes put in place by the Chancellor of the Exchequer, Rishi Sunak, when the pandemic struck the country. The furlough and the job retention schemes have supported a large number of persons through the pandemic. But it is costly and cannot continue for much longer. Hence the Chancellor has announced that furlough would cease in October. The economy needs to improve to help bring in tax revenues. Getting back to work is another matter. The country cannot afford an autumn of lockdown. We are then likely to end in a spiral of national debt like had happened in Greece.

How is this debt going to be paid back as we certainly would have to do in the years to come?

Fortunately the UK was in a good place economically at the start of the pandemic. Public borrowing had come down after the financial crisis of 2008. And currently interest rates are low allowing the government to manage the debt. Also the UK has a good credit rating which allows borrowing on reasonable terms.

However even if the economy recovers, taxes would need to rise to fund services and to bear down on the enormous debt. Having been through almost five years of austerity, any further reductions in services especially in the NHS would be a no-go area for any government. This is made more acute by the reduction in some health services for e.g. in cancer and heart disease during shutdown. These services would now have to be provided and the backlogs managed.

A pandemic is different to a traditional war in that the life has to go on as far as possible as normal but people have to practice physical distancing which is not asked for in war. Even as far as work is concerned, this must continue unabated or even at a greater intensity to support the war effort. Hence manufacturing, food production etc would increase. If these activities ceased during war, the inevitable would follow- loss. On the other hand, in a pandemic physical distancing is a tool used to combat the infection, in the current context the virus, SARSCov2. Therefore government policy on managing the current pandemic is about balancing bearing down on the virus while trying to protect the economy. As there is no effective treatment for or protection against the virus like a vaccine as yet, the only measures that are available are physical distancing, hand washing and the use of face coverings.

In the current pandemic the advice on physical distancing has had the effect of virtually eliminating the work force from the work place when lockdown was instituted on 23rd March. The effect of this was to severely curtail economic activity, which still continues. Closure of schools has added to the diminishing workforce because parents need to be at home to care for children. Carers. grandparents, friends etc are not available to look after children as they too are respecting distancing regulations.

Richard D Smith, Marcus R Keogh-Brown and Tony Barnett, from LSHTM wrote in 2009 about 'prophylactic absenteeism' (PA). This is where a person makes a conscious decision to keep away from work for fear of contracting the infection. It is known that when there is a high fatality rate from the pandemic the incidence of professional absenteeism rises. It also rises when there are deaths in a person's 'effective social network' of family, friends, colleagues etc. Richard Smith and colleagues wrote about the death of someone close becoming 'internalised' and thus contributing to 'professional absenteeism'. PA does not appear to be an issue with the current pandemic because absence from work applied to all except those engaged in providing essential services. However the factors known to affect PA may play a part in delaying return to work in the current climate.

Following the SARS pandemic of 2003, Zia Sadique, John Edmunds and colleagues published in 2007 the results of a survey of people's behaviours to a hypothetical pandemic. The research was conducted in three Asian countries and five countries in Europe, with the UK being one of them. They found that 75% of those who responded would avoid public transport and 30% would confine themselves indoors. In an interesting regional difference they found that Europeans were more likely to avoid places of entertainment while Asians avoided seeing their doctors.

It was estimated that during the SARS pandemic, the economies of southeast Asian countries lost about $60 billion. Considering the likely duration of the current Covid-19 pandemic it is no wonder that the effect on global economies is of a much greater magnitude. It was known in 2007 that pandemic influenza would reduce the UK GDP by up to 10%

In addition to government induced lockdown, personal fear is a potent reason for people to avoid exposure to risk of infection. Research has shown that vaccination may help to reduce the adverse impact of a pandemic on health and also on the economy.

Health economists inevitably ask whether it is worth spending on Covid-19. An evil question but one that has to be asked. It is a question asked every day in health economics. The National Institute of Health and Care Excellence (NICE) in the UK asks this question in all its work. How much would the UK spend on a particular treatment or a drug? Therefore it is natural to ask what the UK would spend on managing the pandemic. It all boils down to a cost versus benefit analysis. For example the ONS said that for the week ending 3 April there were 3475 deaths from Covid-19 in England and Wales but 6082 more deaths from all causes during the same week compared to the average number of deaths for the same week past 5 years. Taking these figures during this specific week one could have a variety of views. The optimist would claim that 3475 deaths due to Covid-19 were avoided by effective and timely treatment. This is tangible and visible. The 6082 excess deaths are a nebulous figures and something held in the minds of statisticians and the like. The pessimist would be extremely unsettled by the unnecessary loss of 6082 lives which were not directly due to Covid-19. He would say these should have been avoided by appropriate separation of and continuation of provision of services for them. This does not take into account that many would not have sought advice from their doctors and would have been reluctant to go to their GP's or hospital for fear on contracting Covid-19. Herein lays the dilemma with numbers. Even if one took the evil and immoral decision not to treat any of the 3475 patients with Covid-19 there is no guarantee that the 6082 lives would have been saved. Individual perceptions of the pandemic may have contributed to delayed diagnosis and treatment contributing to an early death.

Gita Gopinath, from the IMF said 'The Covid-19 pandemic pushed economies into a Great Lockdown, which helped contain the virus and save lives, but also triggered the worst recession since the Great Depression.' She went on to say that 'in the absence of a medical solution, the strength of the recovery is highly uncertain and the impact on sectors and countries uneven.' Living standards were expected to drop in more than 95% of countries.

The IMF expects a 0.2% contraction in GDP which would be worse than in the US, Germany, Japan and Canada. Also it is expected that the UK economy would shrink by 3.7% this year and to rise by 2.3% in 2021. However, as the pandemic spreads it is likely that these projected figures may change. These figures reflect the massive adverse economic impact of Covid-19 in the UK.

Towards the end of April, the Governor of the Bank of England,

Andrew Bailey, maintained that the country needed to move cautiously if it was considering a release from lockdown. He was concerned that too early a release may lead to a spike in infections which in turn would lead to a re-imposition of lockdown regulations. Re-imposition would damage public confidence which could adversely have affected the economy.

There is no doubt that furlough and other financial support measures for the economy and for the workforce was the right thing to do at the time. However none of these measures could last more than a few months. It was therefore not unexpected that the Chancellor, Rishi Sunka, advised that furlough would end in October. Encouraging people, to spend for e.g. by financial support for eating out at restaurants was a means to give people the confidence to go out and spend. It also appeared to have encouraged people to get out, return to work, and to socialise more that they had done for some months. Return to work is necessary with adequate precautions while the impact on the spread of the virus by this and by children returning to schools is being monitored.

The UK is otherwise at risk of having very rapidly, thanks to Covid-19, moved from a country with low-unemployment to one where a significant number are unemployed with even greater cost to the Exchequer.

On 16th June the ONS reported that 600,000 jobs were lost during lockdown. Lord Hague (William Hague, a previous leader of the Conservative Party and Leader of the Opposition) said in response that these job losses 'represent a personal catastrophe for hundreds of thousands of people'. He called the lockdown a 'disaster (that) cannot under any circumstances be repeated'.

However, even if the UK comes out of lockdown there is no possibility of it ever returning to its previous levels of work, entertainment, other social activities etc. Many businesses would have collapsed and many people would be added to the register of those who are unemployed. The cost to the Exchequer of a ballooning unemployment rate would be as great as the spend on supporting the economy during the pandemic. To this cost if one added the costs entailed in having to retrain people for the same or other jobs, one realises that the 'tsunami' of employment would scar the UK economy for a long time. At the start of the pandemic the UK had one of the lowest unemployment rates in the world of 3.6%

Leisure and hospitality appear to be the worst affected sectors of the economy. Social distancing prevented restaurants, pubs and hotel from opening. Even during the gradual easing from lockdown in June these businesses remained closed. The economic output from this sector was below 90% of that which it was in January 2020. The restaurant and hospitality industry claims that almost 40 years of continuing growth came abruptly to a standstill and it is not likely to return to its pre-lockdown levels. Take that sandwich industry as an example. It was started by Marks and Spencer which sold a sandwich in 1980 for just 43p. It has now grown into a ubiquitous presence in every supermarket and corner shop. The range of sandwiches and flavours available were probably unimaginable to the pioneers of the sandwich industry. Every palate is catered for. Glencoe, a company that makes sandwiches produced 700 million packed sandwiches in 2019. That is just a third of the two billion or so sandwiches bought in the UK that year. Some companies are thinking about diversifying their methods of delivery of sandwiches and other foods. It is unlikely that turnover would ever reach previous levels of activity.

Construction was the next worst affected part of the economy with output dropping by 40%. Not surprisingly the communication and information technology sectors were hardly affected. The finance and insurance industries only suffered a 5 % reduction in activity.

The airline industry was severely affected by the pandemic. The government position of using 2- week quarantine for all arrivals into the UK has considerably reduced air travel. At the height of lockdown air traffic plummeted in the UK to 6% of normal activity. With easing of restrictions this figure rose to only 30% of normal flights.

Several MP's, airlines and operators of airports have written to the government to rethink its position about the 14-day quarantine imposed on travellers. Rolls-Royce which builds aircraft engines and which is significantly affected by lockdown also supported a review of the quarantine regime. Its chief executive, Warren East said 'aviation has a vital role to play in helping the world recover from the pandemic and that 'getting people flying again needs to be a high priority for the Government.' It is said that the tourism industry is losing £650 million a week. It was predicted that the travel and tourism industry in UK would lose £20 billion as a result of lockdown.

In June, SAGE had requested Public Health England to consider testing arrivals twice - once on arrival and again five to eight days later. Only a small number of positive cases would be picked up by testing at the time of arrival. This rises to 85% after five days of arrival and to 96% when the test is done eight days after arrival. The policy of serial testing would enable quarantine to be reduced to eight days.

Linda Bauld, professor of public health at the University of Edinburgh of the view that quarantine is a "blunt instrument".

Usually, following a recession the UK economy returns to relatively normal levels after about three years. But this time, the pandemic has brought with it a set of unusual and costly issues like furlough, social distancing and carefully calculated return to work and schools. All these aspects of the pandemic have conspired to place an unusual burden on the economy. It would take a long time to return to a semblance of what is normal. Unemployment would in the meantime continue to increase.

Which brings us back to equipoise. The longer return to work and schools is delayed the economy is near stagnant. The Health and Social Services budget is £140.4 billion for 2019/2020. To continue to maintain this level of spending and to increase annually at least in line with inflation would require the economy to be vibrant. The longer that there is delay in kick-starting the economy, the impact on health is likely to be felt sooner rather than later.

There would have to be a calculated risk accepted by all, in any release form lockdown. There would never be a safe time to come out en-masse from lockdown. It would have to be a slowly managed process. Businesses may clamour for release but it is the government that would bear the financial costs and also be held to account if there are further peaks of the infection. The experience of New Zealand, Germany and some other countries including in the UK shows how the infection could easily slip back into the community unless stringent preventive measures are in place and they are enforced.

o0:0o

AFTERMATH

Covid-19 is a great leveller. No one is immune to it and everyone, without exception, is susceptible to it. Apart from the physical illness, Covid-19 has taught all of us a lot about ourselves. And it has shown us much about the world around us. There can never be true equality of people but it is an aim that all societies and governments, at least in liberal democracies, aspire to. There would always be differences between the rich and the not so rich and between the haves and those that have not.

Why is it that the UK failed whereas countries like South Korea and New Zealand succeeded in containing the pandemic? South Korea which had previously experienced SARS and MERS had a well oiled machine to deal with any impending threat. So when Covid-19 appeared, it instituted widespread testing. By the middle of March 2020 over a quarter of a million people had been tested. Those who tested positive were traced and tracked using mobile phone technology. Tracing of cases was vital in containing the illness and its spread. Most offices and other buildings used by people have heat sensors at the entrances. Anyone found to have a raised temperature was sent for testing to exclude the possibility of Covid 19. All the preventive steps taken by South Korea have allowed the country of nearly 53 million people to have only 10,728 cases of Covid-19 and 242 deaths as of 27th April 2020.

In New Zealand there were 1461 cases of Covid -19 and 18 deaths as of 27th April 2020. New Zealand closed it borders early in the pandemic and introduced social distancing. It was with pride that Jacinda Adern, the

Prime Minister, declared on 26th April 2020 that 'we have won the battle, and stopped community transmission of the disease'.

In contrast, in the UK time appeared to have been wasted. There was conspicuous lack of any meaningful action in February 2020 while there was talk about increasing herd immunity. Herd immunity is a protective concept based on how many people in a group are protected. The larger the number protected, the immunity of the entire herd is higher and the whole group benefits from protection. That is the basis of all immunisation programmes – to achieve as wide coverage as possible, even 100% so that herd immunity is 100% or as far as possible close to this figure. High herd immunity may be achieved by two means. If many people in a group or in a country get a disease that induces protective antibodies and therefore immunity, then herd immunity rises. Therefore to get, say, 90% herd immunity in this way we would need 90% of the group or in the UK, 90% of the population getting the infection. We were repeatedly told that for most persons Covid-19 was a minor illness. If this was so and if the most vulnerable in society were protected or shielded from it, we should have been able to reach high herd immunity, if the vast majority of the others got a mild version of the illness and recovered from it.The alternative course would have been to vaccinate the majority of the population as we do for example with MMR (measles, mumps, rubella). But there was no vaccine against Covid-19. Therefore even the smallest amount of herd immunity was never achievable in the UK unless a significant proportion of the population got the infection.

The isolation of patients, tracing and testing contacts of patients with Covid-19 and general testing of the population linked to quarantine would have been the most effective strategy to contain the virus. We depended on tests, millions of them, bought from China. These were found to be defective. The UK was therefore left with no meaningful or joined-up strategy to combat Covid -19. Germany was able to produce its own tests. Why is the UK not capable of producing its own tests? The UK's dependence for supplies of most things from abroad exposed how vulnerable it is. It was therefore inevitable that the UK had one of the largest number of Covid-19 cases in Europe.

The pandemic showed that the UK needed an essential and important change in its ability to be self sufficient in health supplies as in many other things, like food. Our dependence on services to support the economy has shown to be woefully inadequate. Even if a vaccine was discovered in the UK, its production on a massive scale would, of necessity, have needed to be located abroad. The pharmaceutical firm Astra-Zeneca is working with Oxford University to produce a vaccine against Covid-19. However large –scale production of any successful vaccine would be by the Russian pharmaceutical company, R-Pharm which is located in Moscow. We are then again dependent on the producers and the laws of the producer countries. There is no doubt any producer nation of a vaccine would seek to satisfy the needs of its own nationals first before exporting elsewhere. Altruism is good in times of plenty!

The failure to test for Covid-19 and trace contacts of those who carried the virus contributed in no small way to the spread of the pandemic. Testing was ceased in March 2020 at a time when the country should have been testing and tracing more. It is surprising that the Deputy Chief Medical Officer claimed that testing and tracing was not an effective strategy. However, when testing was started later in the pandemic, it was slow and cumbersome. The advice that led to testing being abandoned in March needs to be re-visited. Similarly the advice to discharge patients from hospital to care homes without testing is now known to have been a significant error. Couple this decision with lack of testing of residents and staff of care homes and there was a recipe for infections and therefore deaths from Covid-19 in care homes.

There needs to be an effective test and trace system which is based locally. It should be operated by local public health departments but remain accountable to a central system. Take the case of the national cervical smear testing program. It is managed by the NHS Screening Committee but the work is done locally in General Practices, gynaecology departments, sexual health clinics etc. supported by local accredited pathology laboratories. There are effective microbiology laboratories attached to each acute hospital which manages all local infections. Scattered around the UK are also several private laboratories which could be used in a crisis. These are the natural sites for testing if there is a second wave or another pandemic in a few years time. To start a test and trace system from scratch and by an organization that has no track record in the process is a recipe for failure. It is unlikely that selection of personnel, their training and deployment countrywide could be done in haste and to expect it to be successful. Review of testing and tracing must be done as a matter of urgency. Testers and tracers could be stood down when demand for their services is low, but have regular updates so that they are readily available if the need arises. One does not get a test and trace system overnight. It comes from years of practice. It would be also useful for the UK to have a hybrid system of Smartphone apps and a manual strategy for tracing contacts of the disease. It is known that the test and trace pilot in the Isle of Wight was hugely successful in reducing the R number on the island. The Isle of Wight was the 147th out of 150 in the ranking of R number in local authorities in mid-April. This dropped to it having the 10th lowest R number at the end of June 2020. Why is it not being used nationally? The advantage of a complementary manual system is the comforting voice of a real human being that can place matters in perspective and assuage fears

Public Health England is a body responsible to the Department of Health, with its role in protecting the health of the public. The advice, during the pandemic, from PHE to the Department of Health and to ministers also needs to be reviewed. There needs to be a root and branch reform of PHE. It appears to have failed significantly in dealing with the pandemic and in protecting the public. There have been calls, and not without reason, that the role of PHE in the health of the nation be reviewed. However any re-organisation of PHE would follow a critical review of its role in the current pandemic and its role in the future. To do otherwise would be yet another Health Service re-organisation in the midst of a pandemic without clear objectives. Lessons have to be learned and changes effected on the basis of evidence. PHE was established in 2013; it has a wide remit in protecting the nation's health. This includes dealing with smoking, the obesity crisis that is affecting the UK and other public health issues. Any discussion about the future of the PHE must take account of funding of the service. In the UK government's Spending Review of 2015, George Osborne, the then Chancellor of the Exchequer said 'This spending review is the next step in our plan to eliminate the deficit, run a surplus and ensure Britain lives within its means.' But Anita Charlesworth who was chief economist at the Health Foundation said that the changes had 'cost the health system dearly'. It was reported that the cuts to NHS funding at the time meant a reduction in UK health spending from 7.3 per cent of GDP in that financial year to just 6.7 per cent. The Health Foundation said that as a result the UK's spending on health was below that of comparable countries like the USA, France and Germany. John Appleby, chief economist at the King's Fund, an independent health care charity that works to improve care in the England, said that whatever additional funding to the NHS was obtained through significant cuts to other Health Department budgets. He said that 'cutting the public health budget is a false economy, undermining the government's commitments on prevention at a time when the need to improve public health is becoming increasingly urgent.' Anita Charlesworth claimed that the government had given with one hand and taken away with the other. This was a 'false economy' and the outlook for health services was 'bleak' and it was a 'false economy'.

The Prime Minister used words like ' shock', 'a nightmare', disaster' during his appearance on radio at the end of June. He said "The country has gone through a profound shock. But in those moments you have the opportunity to change and to do things better. We really want to build back better, to do things differently,…'. Yes the country has been and is still going through a profound shock at the time of this writing. Apart from the whole country being turned upside down there has also been, in the minds of many people, a shock at what had been happening to the country in the past 25 years or so. We realised how vulnerable we are and how dependent we are on the rest of the world. In an interconnected world, a global village, interdependence is a sine qua non. But the extreme dependence we have on the outside world has been a wakeup call. There was clearly 'shock' at seeing that for e.g. the NHS did not have enough ventilators and PPE.

In 1945 John Blease and Drs. Henry Roberts and John Halton devised and manufactured the Blease ventilator. John Blease incidentally also manufactured his 'Blease Special' 1000cc motor cycle in the 1930's. The first known ventilator was the 'iron lung'. It was also called a 'tank ventilator' where the whole human body was placed inside a tank, save for the head. It was first described by a Scottish physician John Dalziel in 1838. The tank ventilator saved the lives of many who suffered with poliomyelitis which had paralysed muscles used in breathing. Subsequently one encountered in UK the Barnet ventilator which was manufactured by a company, W Watson and Son Limited of Barnet, England. This shows that the design and manufacturing expertise was there and still is. Why one may ask, does this manufacturing activity not continue so as to supply the NHS and UK social care? These products would also have been available for export.

Take the case of Harold Horace Hopkins who was a physicist in Reading University. He invented the solid rod lens system which formed the basis of telescopy in medicine. His lens system was patented in 1959. But the patent was bought by Karl Storz of Karl Storz GmbH of Germany, which now manufactures and sells telescopes for use in medicine and in industry. Do we manufacture lenses, telescopes or endoscopes in the UK today?

Or the case of the humble television. John Logie Baird was a Scottish engineer who invented and demonstrated television in 1926. And in 1928 he demonstrated the first transatlantic television transmission. The UK does not now manufacture television sets either.

The same could be said about the motor car, trains, aeroplanes and even the simple bicycle. Why has the UK presided over the near decimation of these industries? The shift of the economy from manufacturing to the service sector must now be seen as a 'shock' with the realisation that these industries have been lost.

Unions also have a vital part to play in the resurrection of manufacturing and services in the UK. Many may remember the strikes at the then British Leyland car manufacturing plants or the problems regarding printing in Fleet Street and the strikes that followed. Without attempting to pass judgement on the rights or wrongs of these events, about which much has been written, the important lesson here is that their needs to be a meeting of minds between employer and employee. There is no doubt that unions are needed to protect the rights of individuals in the workplace and to ensure that safe, dignified working conditions exist. By the same token unions have a responsibility to their members, to the employer or company and to the public. Unions should not be used as political tools to achieve political ends, nor should unions be seen to act in such a manner. Employers for their part need to recognise the immense value that employees bring to the success of the organisation or company and employers need to ensure that there are reasonable working conditions. The pursuit of profits and dividends should not be the sole purpose of a company. Good customer service and employee protection would ensure the continued health of a company.

The loss of the manufacturing base in the UK has had grave repercussions for employees and their families. If a company has to shut as is likely to occur due to the coronavirus pandemic, then it becomes the duty of government to help save as many jobs as possible and to provide support, training and re-deployment for those who would lose their jobs.

Even the nation's utilities are owned by foreign companies. In one ten year period the water companies made about £18 billion in profit. Less than one billion pounds of this money was invested in the service, mainly infrastructure repairs and updates. One of the biggest losses of water in the UK are from leaking water mains. The rest of the profit was paid as dividends to shareholders. And we heard appeals from water companies about conserving water during the pandemic. This was apparently due to increased consumption of water by people staying at home during lockdown. It is always a source of amazement to have heard that privatised utilities would be able to source the necessary funds to invest in the respective companies. But what one sees is the vast majority of profits are paid to shareholders while the companies are indebted to banks. This is an unusual business model which places the taxpayer always at risk. To the average person all of this does not make any logic. Why not use the profits to pay down the debts owed by the water companies? Why not use a greater slice of the profits in improving the water supply infrastructure? Why not use some of the profits to bear down on household bills? There is a regulator, Ofwat, Water Services Regulatory Authority, which appears unable to influence decisions made by water companies. Can Ofwat be said therefore to be acting in the interest of the customer? Change should occur and there is no better time than now. This is a time for taking stock and government needs to step in to prevent this manner of profit taking or the way companies are run with debt but simultaneously paying out excessive dividends. Why cannot the government rule that not more than, say, 50% of profits may be paid as dividends to shareholders? And make it mandatory for companies to pay off debts and invest in infrastructure and better service to customers.

For too long we have sat silently while witnessing some of the UK's best talents and businesses being sold to outsiders who have no interest in the UK. Their sole purpose is to 'steal' knowledge and technology from the UK. The chocolate manufacturer, Cadburys was taken over by Kraft Foods in 2010. There was much public opposition to the sale of Cadburys. The advisers for the takeover were UBS, Goldman Sachs and Morgan Stanley who made considerable amounts in fees. Probably the most controversial participant in the sale was the Royal Bank of Scotland (RBS) which provided the funds to Krafts. RBS faced collapse in 2008 and was bailed out by the UK government, which owned 84% of RBS. In 2007 Boots the Chemist was bought by the private investment firm Kohlberg Kravis Roberts and Stefano Pessina. Many of the water utilities are privately owned with only limited amounts of profits being invested in the companies. The UK is a world leader in digital technology. The company Imagination Technologies designs and manufactures graphic chips for Apple computers. Imagination Technologies started life in 1985 and was listed on the London Stock Exchange in 1994. Apple planned to acquire Imagination Technologies but instead eventually in 2017 it stopped using Imaginations' intellectual property on its chips. Imagination's stock price fell by 70% and eventually the company was sold to private equity company, Canyon Bridge which was owned by the government of China. Since this sale took place there have been security concerns about technology transfers to China. Global Counsel, a public affairs company of which Peter Mandelson is chairman had links with Canyon Bridge. The managing director of Global Counsel had apparently advised Canyon Bridge on how it should respond to inquiries by the UK Foreign Affairs Select Committee. That many who had authority when in power in the UK government appeared to work against the interest of the UK is worrying. Global Counsel maintained that it advised Canyon Bridge on 'policy matters relating to its investment portfolio', whatever this may mean. With the issues relating to Huawei it is natural for the government to look again at risks to national security. The Chairman of the Foreign Affairs Committee, Tom Tugendhat, wrote that the actions of some persons are 'immoral, unjust and un-British'. The former Prime Minister, Harold Macmillan likened the sale of state assets to 'selling the family silver'. But what has happened in recent years is a sale of assets, some of which are important for national security. It seems important that the majority stake in some companies must be in British possession.

As Clive Hamilton wrote it is important for the UK to extricate itself from involvement with China. This is especially so where infrastructure, industries, technology etc are concerned. He wrote that 'greed, naivety and complacency' by decision makers have allowed China to gain a foothold in many aspects of British life. Those who facilitated and encouraged this trend are truly China's useful idiots.

For too long the UK has been prepared to sell its brains and its brawns to the highest bidder. For too long the country has allowed corporate greed and personal enrichment to dominate the economic landscape of the country.

This is the moment of change for the UK. Our industrial failings have been exposed, like our lack of preparedness for the pandemic. The Prime Minister appears determined to get the country and its economy back to normal. What better time to bring about a change in the UK's approach to its economy?

Why is the UK not producing ventilators, PPE and all the other consumer goods, from toys to cars that it used to produce? Why do companies and employees supinely accept the status quo when all that is invented or co-invented in the UK is lost abroad? Covid-19 has turned an important dictum of Adam Smith on its head. Adam Smith was a Scottish, philosopher and author who is considered the 'Father of Economics'. He was a champion and, in effect, the first prophet of the free market. In 1776 in his book 'An Inquiry in the Nature and Causes of the Wealth of Nations', Adam Smith wrote 'In every country it always is and must be the interest of the great body of the people to buy whatever they want of those who sell it cheapest. The proposition is so very manifest that it seems ridiculous to take any pains to prove it..'. However, the pandemic has exposed the vulnerable underbelly of this dictum of capitalism. When faced with a crisis, the 'each one for himself' principle immediately comes into play. Countries quite naturally forgot global altruism and looked after their own populations. Politicians are after all accountable to their public, not to the world. See how Germany did not allow ventilators to be sent to Italy at a time when it was at the height of its crisis and despite increasing numbers of deaths. India limited the export of a whole host of medicines including paracetamol and various antibiotics. It was in April that India permitted the export of paracetamol and hydroxychloroquine, with the Ministry of External Affair stating that "given the enormity of the COVID-19 pandemic, India has always maintained that the international community must display strong solidarity and cooperation'. But at the same time India's view is that like any responsible government, India's first obligation is to ensure that there are adequate supplies of medicines for its own people.

India's words and actions and those of Germany for e.g. show why it is vital that the UK has its own supplies.

The news in early July 2020 was that the US had bought up virtually all of the next three months of production of a drug shown to work against Covid-19. The US Department of Health and Human Services (HHS) said it had secured more than 500,000 treatment courses of remdesivir for American hospitals. Remdesivir is an anti-viral drug that was developed for use against Ebola. It has been shown to have some beneficial effect against Covid-19. It is licensed for use in the UK also. The cost of a course of treatment with remdesivir in Covid-19 is said to be about £1900. Prof. Peter Horby from the University of Oxford who is also chairman of NERVTAG raised important ethical questions when he talked about fair access to the drug at a fair price. Tests on the drug were done in the US, Europe and Mexico among other countries. Prof. Horby pointed to the ethical issues related to how participants in trials of the drug would feel if access to it were restricted by the bulk purchase by US, thereby denying others of access to it. Participants in trials of the drug would have done so for altruistic reasons, as often is the case with most drug trials.

The action by the US is not dissimilar to it trying to buy any vaccines for Covid-19. About twenty years ago the US was also trying to purchase large amounts of treatments like the antibiotic, ciprofloxacin, when its citizens were in receipt of letters containing anthrax spores. Some readers may remember two senators, Tom Daschle and Patrick Leahy, who were in receipt of these so called 'anthrax letters'. Following these events and the fear they generated, the US National Strategic Stockpile began accumulating antibiotics and anti-anthrax serum. Fortunately for the UK there are adequate supplies of remdesivir, if the need arises.

Stockpiling of drugs and material by a country for use by its citizens is as understandable as it is reasonable. But countries also need to have responsibility for the rest of the world. What we have seen with the coronavirus pandemic is a degree of 'national selfishness' with drugs, ventilators etc.

Ensuring supply chains for essential medicines and emerging drugs is vital during any future pandemic or any other threats to public health. Stockpiling of medicines is prudent practice. But when a country seeks to commandeer total production of essential medicines, other governments are compelled to act to ensure supply for their citizens. The Netherlands and Australia considered suspending patent laws to allow others companies to manufacture essential drugs. This is a step of last resort, but must be considered carefully when it appears that a medicine is likely to be needed. In this context it is useful to think about the use of the drug dexamethasone in Covid-19. It was found to be useful in patients with Covid-19 who are on ventilation in intensive care and needed oxygen. Dexamethasone is a cheap medicine. But there have been examples in the past where very cheap medicines have suddenly gone up in price when demand increases or alternative uses are found for a drug. Here again, in the face of a grave threat to the public, a government must be able to seek powers to ensure supplies of medicines at a fair price, while being mindful of the need of other countries.

The UK contributed to many of the inventions in the world in the twentieth century, especially in the first half of the last century. It is time that the UK returned to its industrial heritage. By reclaiming our industrial past the UK would not only be more self reliant but also, with its basic humanitarianism, it could be a force for good in the world. As the country embarks on a new course after Brexit, it could show itself as a vibrant, neo-industrial nation. Many may scoff at the thought that the UK has a moral basis for its actions, or indeed that it even has any degree of morality left. Morality is not a perfect art or science. But the UK could still claim to act morally in many, often difficult, situations.

The pandemic has given the world an insight into China and its modus operandi within China and around the word. One has only to look at the industrial and financial power of China. China combines this power with a basic lack of morality and decency. Take the example of its treatment of the Uighur population who live in an autonomous region in north-west China. Uighur people are forced to have sterilisations, abortions and the insertion of intra-uterine contraceptive devices in women to prevent pregnancy.

China's determination to cut the birth rate among Uighurs has generated a feeling of terror among the population. China of course denies that all this is happening while at the same time building detention centres for the Uighurs in the name of 're-education'. At other times China does not deny its actions, which it claims are needed to control religious extremism in the country. This is a glaring example of the duplicity of Chinese talk, for at the same time it claims that reports of mistreatment of Uighurs are fake news. Some writers claim that the large scale internment of the Uighurs is the largest incarceration of an ethno-religious group since the holocaust. Other writers do not stop short of calling the activities of the Chinese regime as genocide. Then again we have had examples of evidence of prison labour in goods arriving from China. China's claims to the contrary are in stark contrast to its actions. It is one of the most repressive regimes in the world which tightly controls its citizens. It seems that control in this context applies to even control of thought. The UK on the contrary can be proud of its freedoms.

It is not surprising that at the UN Human Right's Council, 53 countries supported China in its current crackdown in Hong Kong but there was no mention of what is happening to China's Uighur population. It is not surprising that the USA pulled out of the UN's Human Rights Council calling it a 'cesspool of political bias' and that it was a 'hypocritical' body that 'makes a mockery of human rights'.

China's approach to the rest of the world is nothing short of aggressive, coupled with double speak. It was about July that the UK government was seriously considering whether to allow the Chinese telecommunication company, Huawei, a stake in the non-core parts of the UK's 5G telecommunications networks. There initially appeared to be an agreement in principle to allow Huawei a 30% stake in UK's 5G networks. The decision to allow this to proceed was being seriously re-considered by the government with some pressure from the USA. There were concerns expressed by the US and UK security services that there could be breaches of UK security if Huawei was allowed to operate in the country. This prompted the Chinese Ambassador in the UK, Liu Xiaoming, to suggest that any reversal of the decision would damage the view, in China, of the UK as a country that is open for business. He warned that if the UK treated China as a hostile country, there would be consequences that would follow. He did not specify what these consequences were. He may have been referring to trade between the two countries. He however implied that Chinese business may not be able to trust the UK. The US ambassador in the UK said that trust in Huawei cannot exist as it is a company that is answerable to the Chinese government and the Chinese Communist Party.

During the pandemic Chinese banks were ordered to use part of their profits amounting to £171 billion by to lower lending rates so as to help the economy recover. The Governor of the People's Bank of China, Yi Gang, said 'Financial institutions are urged to sacrifice profits to benefit corporate borrowers, helping reducing their borrowing costs'. This is a step banks in the UK could follow. But the important operative word here is 'urged'. The Chinese banks would have to do as 'urged'. For the word 'urged' read 'ordered'. Banks, like all businesses including Huawei, are not independent of the government. They would, in the final analysis, have to do as they are 'urged'.

Following cancellation of the Huawei deal, the China Global Times newspaper reported that 'it is necessary for China to retaliate against the UK – otherwise wouldn't we be too easy to bully. Such retaliation should be public and painful for the UK'. The Chinese ambassador in the UK talked about fairness and openness and the need for the UK to be non-discriminatory. The former Foreign Secretary, Lord Hague was sufficiently concerned to warn the UK not to be dependent on China for technology because it did not 'play by our rules'.

Seldom, must there have been an occasion when a vendor has threatened a purchaser for not buying its wares as the Chinese seems to do after the UK reversed its decision to purchase Hauwei.

Talking about consequences, one may recall the massive cyber attack that Australia endured in the weeks after it called for an investigation on how China had handled the virus infection and how it had shared information with the WHO. China denied any involvement in these attacks on Australia's infrastructure.

At the same time that the UK government was considering how it would deal with Huawei, China unanimously passed a law that would allow it to crack down on protestors in Hong Kong. This was seen as the boldest move yet by China to break down the separation between the

Aftermath

democratic system in Hong Kong and the autocratic communist regime in mainland China. The passage of the law was seen by the UK, USA and many other countries as a move to extend Communist control over Hong Kong. The law would allow China to extradite or imprison persons that it sees as a threat to the Communist Party. In response the US considered withdrawing the preferential trade status that Hong Kong had enjoyed. The law came into effect on 1st July 2020. While the Chinese ambassador in London talked about trust, this was a clear breach of the trust between UK and China when the one country-two systems of government were enshrined in the Basic Law on 1st July 1997. This was the date when Hong Kong was formally handed back to China after one hundred years of British rule.

Many people may not have heard of the 48 Group Club. The headquarters of the club are in London. It is a pro-China organisation dedicated to influencing people in the British establishment. The previous UK Prime Minster, Tony Blair, gave a speech to the club but there is no evidence of him having had any association with the club. Jack Straw the previous Labour Home Secretary on the other had received an honorary fellowship from the club. It is not possible at this stage to know if 48 Group Club has any connection with the Chinese Communist Party or the government of China. Or is it just an organisation helping with an appreciation of China by the West?

A more worrying aspect of China's projection of its politics is the use of its students who are studying in UK universities. The Chinese ambassador in UK, Liu Xiaoming, has urged Chinese students in the UK to be patriotic and to serve the motherland. Chinese students are monitored by the Chinese embassy which uses its own students to spy on fellow students. They are encouraged to further Chinese views and China's interests. Chinese students are encouraged to support China's views on matters of international interest. Healthy debate is suppressed by the sheer numbers of Chinese students who could for e.g. vote to object to the presence of a speaker with an alternative point of view. How many leaders or diplomats have invoked the motherland when speaking to their compatriots? It reminds one of the novel 'Fatherland' by the writer Robert Harris.

The ability of China to manipulate decision making in government departments and in other institutions is a worrying trend which the government of the UK and elsewhere are belatedly waking up to. China attempts to interfere with and to manipulate anything that it perceives as anti- Chinese or which is not in its interests.

On 30th July 2020 the first elected President of Taiwan, Lee Teng-hui died at the age of 97 years. He steered Taiwan from military law to become a vibrant democracy and one of the most successful in Asia. Mainland China which always claimed Taiwan as an integral part of it called Lee Teng-hui 'scum of the nation', a 'secessionist' and a 'traitor' despite him having helped establish trade and economic links with mainland China. Lee Teng-hui was called 'Mr. Democracy' and the US Secretary of State, Mike Pompeo called him a 'beacon of democracy'. China's failure or inability to see the benefits of Taiwan and Hong Kong and its desire to crush democracy shows that its only desire is to retain control by the CCP by all means possible. It is incapable of existing and working peacefully with its neighbours. It recent conflict with India is a case in point. So also its claim to the Senhakus islands which are administered by Japan. China has borders with about 14 countries and has disputes with most of them.

US Health Secretary Alex Azar visited Taipei, the capital of Taiwan in late August and said that 'Taiwan's response to COVID-19 has been among the most successful in the world, and that is a tribute to the open, transparent, democratic nature of Taiwan's society and culture' For her part, President Tsai Ing-wenShe of Taiwan thanked the US for supporting Taiwan's bid to join the WHO from which had been excluded for several years at the behest of China. It is interesting to note what Alex Azar said on the visit –"Taiwan knew very early on ... to not trust some of the assertions coming out of there (Beijing) or validation from the World Health Organization, China as is customary warned the US 'not to play with fire'.

On 31st August the Czech Senate speaker, Milos Vystrcil, visted Tawian to promote business links. He said that the Czech Republic would not accept Beijing's objections to the visit. The Chinese government responded in its usual manner by saying that the Chinese would make 'make him pay a heavy price for his short-sighted behaviour and political opportunism'.

Appeasement seldom works!

Since the start of the pandemic China has engaged in attacking several countries around the world. When the Australian Prime Minister, Scott Morrison, called for an independent inquiry into the pandemic, China's ambassador in Australia, Cheng Jingye, said that Chinese tourists may boycott the country and that his compatriots in China may boycott Australian goods. It is unlikely that the average Chinese consumer would boycott foreign goods that they like unless they are being coerced to do so. The Global Times newspaper compared Australia to 'chewed gum on the bottom of a shoe'.

Chinese people are not averse to attacking their own people for purchasing or appearing to own foreign goods. This is covert coercion.

The Chinese Embassy in Sweden attacked journalists for 'ideological attacks' against China. The Chinese ambassador in Sweden chillingly stated that 'we treat our friends with fine wine but for our enemies we use shotguns'. Of course there is a difference in approach, ideological or not, between the manner in which China conducts itself and how many countries in the rest of world act. But for a country that serves as a permanent member of the United Nations to threaten another country portrays China at its lowest, if not at its worst.

At the start of the pandemic China accused France of not acting in a timely manner in containing the infection. It also accused France of making racist slurs against Dr.Tedros. Finally China accused French care home workers of 'letting residents die of disease and starvation'. The EU produced a report documenting how China continued to 'run a global disinformation campaign to deflect blame for outbreak of the pandemic and to improve its international image'. It appears that China threatened the EU leading to dilution of wording in the report. This is an indictment of the impartiality of the EU and its weakness in not standing up to Chinese pressure. This is in marked contrast to the posture of the USA in this respect. The EU Parliamentary Security and Defence Committee made it known that any altering of the report should not have happened and assured that it 'will never happen again'.

It appears that Chinese officials are out-performing each other by the ugliness of their language. Much of this behavior arises from the education system in China which has been completely overhauled in recent times to portray the country as a victim at the hands of foreigners who invaded China in the last century. The protests in Tiananmen

Square alarmed the CCP. The CCP was witnessing what was happening in the former Soviet Union. There, Mikhail Gorbachev had succeeded the late Konstatin Chernenko as President of the Soviet Union on 11th March 1985. Gorbachev proceeded with the two essential pillars of his governing policy – glasnost and perestroika. By Glasnost he wanted more consultative government to replace the central command and control system of government. In perestroika he sought economic change and the end to central planning. The CCP watched these developments with alarm and interpreted protests in Beijing's Tiananmen Square as a challenge to its authority. Glasnost is anathema to the CCP. Hence the crackdown on the protestors in the Square and the ensuing massacre that followed on 4th and 5th June 1989. To avoid going the same way as the communist countries of Eastern Europe and the previous USSR, the CCP proceeded to re-educate people, especially students. History books were re-written. Education now inculcates in students a hatred of all things foreign and that only the Chinese version of events is the right one. Diversity of opinion or healthy inquiry is not permitted and may be punishable. Peter Purdue who taught Chinese history at the Massachusetts Institute of Technology wrote to Chinese students to say 'they had violated fundamental academic norms of civil discourse and respect. As future leaders of China, they had a responsibility to open their minds, in order to make China strong, and not to indulge in destructive narrow-minded self-righteous indignation'.

Avoidance of national humiliation is the key objective of Chinese national and foreign policy. However looking at the way the CCP conducted itself during the pandemic, it has successfully managed to heap humiliation upon itself. History would yet again judge China harshly.

During the pandemic it has insulted many countries around the world. It seeks to impose its will with rudeness, poor language and a thuggish outlook which seem to say 'you can be friends with us only on our terms'.

That China is a permanent member of the UN or that it serves on the UN Human Rights Council is a travesty.

What the world sees from China is rudeness and thug-like behaviour masquerading as international diplomacy.

As has been written, it is time for a conscious decoupling of countries from China. Those countries, and there are many, who share the democratic values of freedom of opinion and expression, human rights etc have some serious thinking ahead of them in order to preserve the rules-based order of world affairs.

The WHO has been partial in its dealings with China as seen, among other things, by its acceptance of the Chinese position that Taiwan should not play any part in the WHO. Taiwan has managed the pandemic remarkably well by acting quickly on cases and by effective testing and tracking. With a population of over 23 million people it had only 447 cases of Covid -19 at the time of writing and only seven deaths. These numbers are particularly impressive given the geographical proximity of Taiwan to mainland China and the frequent transport links between the two countries. The WHO denied itself the information on how Taiwan coped with the pandemic. Even Prime Minster Shinto Abe of Japan commented that it was regrettable than Taiwan was not allowed to even be an observer at WHO. This is surprising given that the WHO is responsible for global health. It has apparently succumbed to pressure from China to exclude Taiwan and in so doing it has acted against its own founding principle of 1948 that 'health is a human right and all people should enjoy the highest standard of health'. If the WHO is responsible for global health but excludes one section of it, however relatively small, one is entitled to ask if it upholds the 'highest standards of heath' for the entire world.

Taiwan sent an e-mail to the WHO on 31st December 201 about cases of pneumonia and possible human-to-human transmission of the infection. Taiwan did not receive a reply and accused the WHO of a dereliction of duty. The WHO responded by saying that there was no inquiry from Taiwan about human-to-human transmission. Taiwan had told the WHO about isolation of sick people. One cannot escape the conclusion that the WHO did not heed the warning implicit in the email of 31st December 2019 or chose to ignore it. In so doing it placed the health of the world's population at risk, again contradicting its founding principles.

The bias of WHO against Taiwan and in favour of China can be seen in the interview which its employee, Bruce Aylward, assistant Director–General had with the journalist Yvonne Tong from the Hong Kong broadcaster, RTHK, in March 2020. She asked him if the WHO would consider admitting Taiwan to the organization. Bruce Aylward initially claimed he could not hear her and finally hung up on her. This is nothing short of information dictatorship where the employees of the WHO are prevented from responding to a legitimate question. Taiwan has one of the most advanced healthcare systems in the world and the world has much to learn from Taiwan about how it dealt with the pandemic. Taiwan has one of the best Covid-19 statistics and the world's public has the right to know how Taiwan contained the pandemic. Unfortunately Taiwan's Covid-19 statistics are mixed up with China's and published as a single set of figures. That this is grossly unfair to the government and people of Taiwan is obvious. The world has the right to expect the WHO to use all available information, knowledge and skills in dealing with this and future pandemics. What would the WHO do if an infection originates from Taiwan? The world has to wake up to China's belligerence and stand firm against it.

The EU's much valued freedom of movement of people between member countries was stress tested with the onset of the pandemic. This fundamental principle of the EU could not and indeed did not withstand the test! It is the jewel in the crown of the EU which facilitates the free movement of people and goods between the member states. In a similar way that individual countries erected barriers during the recent migrant crisis, this time again each country of the EU acted on its own to protect its citizens. Alarmed by how the pandemic was unfolding in Italy it was natural that national leaders acted in the way they did by closing their borders. One therefore witnessed a closure of boundaries and restrictions imposed on the movement of essential medical supplies outside national boundaries. The constituent parts of the EU gravitated to nation states. This was a real challenge to the EU and showed that the EU was yet again incapable of acting in concert to deal with issues which are of importance to the EU and all of its citizens. The interest of the EU was overridden by national interest. In the middle of June 2020 the EU appealed to countries of the bloc to lift restrictions on the movement of people. The EU's commissioner for home affairs, Ylva Johansson, said that while the situation in relation to Covid-19 was improving, Europe's Centre for Disease Prevention and Control (ECDC) had reported "that having internal border restrictions is not an effective measure". This statement does not stand up to scrutiny as countries around the world introduced social distancing rules. Closure of national boundaries augmented social distancing rules and helped prevent spread of the virus. As they saw other

Aftermath

countries batten down the hatches in the face of the spreading pandemic, the public in each country would have expected their respective politicians to act speedily to protect themselves too. The European public did not and would not have looked to the EU for guidance or action. This is a fundament and primeval response of people throughout the ages. This is what we witnessed in Germany's approach to protecting its citizens. It is therefore not surprising that not all EU countries are equally keen on opening their national borders. There may have been suspicion in some capitals of Europe that not all their national neighbours were as stringent as they had been in bearing down on the pandemic or likely to have been as vigilant thereafter in preventing recurrence of the infection.

Even while the pandemic was raging and some nations of the EU were closing their borders others looked aside as migrants and asylum seekers travelled northwards through Europe to reach Calais. This was the route taken by migrants and asylum seeker s to reach the UK. Among the many migrant are undoubtedly genuine asylum seekers fleeing terror, persecution, fear etc. They would be happy to be in any country of the EU compared to whence they came from. It is generally agreed that a person seeks asylum in the first country he or she sets foot on. It is not meant to be a stepping stone to elsewhere. But what we have witnessed in recent years is the migration of people, in the guise of free movement, northwards across Europe. This is nothing short of institutionalised human trafficking.

Italy had particular reason to feel very badly let down by Europe. During the migration crisis, Italy's Foreign Minister at the time, Angelino Alfano, said that Europe had 'abandoned' Italy. Elisabeth Braw, in the journal Foreign Policy, wrote at the time that the EU is 'abandoning Italy in its hour of need'. Italy did not get the support it needed during the pandemic either. While trying to procure face masks it hit a blank wall by France and Germany. France requisitioned its supply, while Germany banned export of masks. These actions were against the EU principle that ensured free movement of goods. What must have been particularly galling for the Italians at their time of desperation was to learn that France had seized a consignment of four million masks that was partly intended for Italy and Spain. Italy was in a desperate position with the pandemic. The number of deaths was such that coffins had to be lined up in churches. Even the sight of this was not sufficient to move the Germans towards helping their neighbour. The Italian newspaper La Republica referred to Europe as 'Ugly Europe'.

Therefore two of the four freedoms of the EU, freedom of movement of people and of goods were openly flouted by France and Germany. It appears somewhat perverse for the EU to speak about the four freedoms- of people, goods, services and capital- in discussions with UK regarding Brexit. They were anything but sacred freedoms during the pandemic.

One commentator wrote that Europe is dead, but it just cannot recognise it.

What Covid-19 had shown was that when confronted with a crisis, countries of the EU would revert to acting in accordance with statehood. Politicians are responsible to the people of their own countries and not to the EU or to the world. Politicians acted in accordance with what was written by Cicero 'Salus populi suprema lex esto' translated as 'The health of the people should be the supreme law'. The philosopher, John Locke, said of Cicero's statement that it is a basic rule for any government. Why would any country of the EU choose to act differently and against the interest of its own citizens?

Try telling France that it did not win the Football World Cup in 2018, but that it was won by Europe!

A similar variety of opinions were seen in how the EU planned to respond to the economic impact of the coronavirus. The French President Emmanuel Macron and German Chancellor Angela Merkel had agreed to a 500 billion-euro ($543 billion) fund for recovery in the EU following the pandemic. But four countries in northern Europe, Denmark, Austria, the Netherlands and Sweden opposed this plan which involved making grants to countries. The group of four northern countries preferred that these payments be made as loans to those countries. As often happened in the history of the EU, this was a Franco-German plan, but Chancellor Merkel pleaded with the EU bloc of countries to 'present a united front in the world. Several commentators and writers have talked of the EU as a Franco-German construct which has arisen from their shared traumatic history of the last century. This appears to have some credence when one considers that plans for discussion by the EU not invariably follow a meeting of the leaders of the two countries. Some plans may not always be in the interest of every country. This alone is a potent reason for the UK to be out of the EU.

As the UK completes the process of extracting itself from the European Union, it would seem to be an opportune time to reflect on the various issues that affect the EU and its unity as a single entity. It is possible that the UK could have a successful working relationship with the EU as indeed the countries of the EU themselves have independently had with it during the Covid-19 period.

No description of Covid-19 would be complete without some consideration of the ethics and morality of dying. Peter Saul is an intensive care specialist form Newcastle, Australia. In 2013 he talked about dying in the twenty –first century and about how we deal with the terminal stages of life. He talked about the intensive care unit as a place where life is not being saved but a place where death is delayed for another day. What is interesting and important, especially to the lay public, is the ability to recognise when a human being is in the declining stages of life, which may extend for some years. This group of people are not about to die. On the contrary, life may continue for quite some time but at a lower level of functioning compared to their previous active selves.

The impression of 'old age' is largely influenced by the culture in which the topic is being discussed. For e.g. in developed countries old age may be considered to commence when a person reaches the age of 65 years. The United Nations considers 65 years as the onset of old age. However it is not possible to set a definite cut-off age for any definition of the onset of old age. Human progression and development would change the age of onset of old age especially in developing countries. In Africa, 55 years was considered as the beginning of old age. This age would change with advancements in health care, quality of life, increases in longevity etc. The study of ageing is called gerontology and those professionals who care for this group of persons are called geriatricians or geriatric physicians or physicians in the care of the elderly. Gerontologists recognise three groups in old age - the young old (60 to 69), the middle old (70 to 79), and the very old (80+). There are, of course, variations of this classification which recognise that there are many people in early 'old age' who live productive lives although they may have retired from their professions or jobs.

Paul Higgs is Professor of Sociology at University College London and Chris Gilleard is a research fellow at the University of Bath and at University College London. In their book 'Rethinking Old Age' the concept of a fourth age is introduced and discussed. This stage of a person's life obviously merges from the end of the 'third age'. The fourth age of a person is characterised by increasing frailty, helplessness and resulting dependence and increasing episodes of illness. Many persons at this stage in their lives still have active mental capacity and some of them may feel a sense of failure arising from memories of their previous active selves. This of itself may be a cause for withdrawal and depression, which adds to the increasing frailty of the person. There is no specific chronological age at which one would say a person is in the fourth stage of their life. Take the cases of some of the oldest marathon runners. Ken Jones who is eighty-six years old has run every London Marathon since the event started in 1981. Or the world's oldest marathon runner, Fauja Singh, from Ilford in the UK. He ran the Hong Kong marathon when he was 101 years old. He is now 104 years old. Ronald Reagan was 69 years old when he became President of the United States of America. He served two consecutive four year terms as President. During his time in office, President Reagan modernised US nuclear arms. He also worked with the President of the USSR, Mikhail Gorbachev to launch the Strategic Arms Reduction Treaty (START). And of course there is Colonel Tom Moore, the most recent and relevant example of active life in old age.

Ken Jones said that the second half of a marathon is "mind over matter". This statement shows that mind and body can function well into advanced chronological age. The fourth stage of life is reached when physical and mental faculties progressively diminish.

What then is the 'third stage' in a person's life? The third stage arose from the *Universités du Troisième Âge* or the University of the Third Age which was started by Prof. Pierre Vellas in Toulouse in 1973. The British historian Peter Laslett wrote about the four ages of man. He described the third stage as a time when a person has retired from their regular job or occupation, but retains good health and remains active, both physically and mentally. The third stage follows from the second stage of increasing maturity and independence.

It is obvious Peter Saul was referring to the fourth age in his talk. Early recognition of the fourth stage of life is important to help elicit and so carry out the wishes of the person before they become too frail and unable to do so. It is vital to ascertain the wishes of the person about the terminal stages of life. In its absence, decisions are then left to family who may not always represent the wishes of the person. These are difficult conversations. But it is important to have these discussions with the person when they are able to make a meaningful contribution. Hard as they are, these distressing conversations help to set the scene for care when increasing frailty of the fourth age sets in. What do you want done Dad, if you are so ill that you are unable to decide yourself or you are unable to communicate to us your wishes? A simple straightforward question but often difficult to set in train a conversation that would lead to this question. But when had, the conversation provides answers that are likely to ease suffering in the terminal stage of life. The term 'suffering' includes the prolonging of life which is only an existence devoid of any semblance of quality. How often have we heard the words 'I lost my mum months ago' or 'she is no more the person we knew as our mum'.

It is possible and indeed imperative to replace the heroic and futile interventions in the terminal days and weeks of life with humane care and compassion. Many people have a lonely mechanised existence provided by life- maintaining equipment which at most would extend 'life' or more accurately extends existence for a short period. Would it not be better to be surrounded by loved ones and to have a duration of life with quality, rather than a marginally longer 'existence' devoid of any quality. As Peter Saul says this is not an advertisement for euthanasia. It is an appeal for compassion during a person's final journey. We have to question whether a needless extension of existence is what our loved ones would have wanted?

The vast majority of people would go through the fourth stage of life. It is characterised by gradually diminishing functions of various body systems- bones and joints affected with arthritis, muscle wasting and weakness causing difficulty in standing and walking, poor vision and hearing, increased risks of falls, neuro-degenerative disease like Parkinsons Disease, Alzheimer's and other types of dementia etc. The human body is comparable to a complex machine. The day arrives when the various systems that keep the human body functioning gradually begin to fade. And with each failing system there is not an additive reduction in duration of remaining life. There is an exponential contraction in the available life span. An important system failure is the ability to resist infection, and to defend oneself from attack by germs of various types. The cumulative effects of chronic diseases, advancing age and frailty leads inevitably to reduced function and eventually death. That is how the majority of people are likely to die. Any event like a heart attack, chest infection etc could be the straw that breaks the camel's back and tips the person into an irretrievable stage of decline and eventual death. Does one intervene heroically to buy a few days of life or act humanely to provide a decent passage during the final journey? It is said that 60% of people in Miami, USA die in intensive care units. Is this where most of us would choose to die? Separated from our families and friends, connected to machines, long removed from reality, the person is in a limbo state which eventually ceases when machines are switched off. The person ceased to be the person they were, many days or even weeks previously. Why? Because someone in the family said 'I want everything possible done for him'. 'Everything possible' can be done. Medicine has the technology to keep the heart beating and the lungs breathing. Drugs can keep the circulation flowing through the body but life departed many days ago and with it the person. Existence continues, but with no meaning to it. What it is to be human was lost on the way? What is sadly left is a de-humanised existence. Why then do we allow our loved ones to descend into such a state just for a few more days, devoid of any quality or any sense of living in the real meaning of the word?

Would not any reasonable person choose to spend the last days of his or her life surrounded by family in the familiar surroundings of home?

Nothing in the preceding paragraphs should be taken to imply that meaningful and necessary treatment must not be provided to all those who need it. On the contrary, the futility of extending life devoid of any quality needs to be given serious consideration.

Those persons who are terminally ill and clearly in the final phase of decline are the group that Peter Saul talked about. The philosophical dilemma here is whether everything possible must be done to save life. The natural answer would be a resounding 'yes'. How often has one heard a family asking that 'everything possible' be done to save a loved one? This is a natural human reaction; it is an appeal reflecting a real human need to preserve life of a loved one. It transcends all cultures. This is not to say that appropriate treatment and care should be denied someone who is ill.

But there comes a time when one would conclude, on behalf of a loved one that he or she has had enough. 'There comes a time when you have to choose between turning the page or closing the book'. And the crux of the matter is whose choice it is to turn the page or to close the book. The discussion about choice would ideally have been had with the person at a stage when they would have been free to express their wishes and were able to clearly articulate their reasons for them.

It is in this time of diminishing function which includes reducing physical, mental and social functioning that one encounters a discussion with the medical profession about mental capacity. The purpose of these discussions is to elicit whether a person is able to make meaningful decisions about their life and its continuation. In the absence of mental capacity one would have to resort to a Power of Attorney. Prior discussions would help avert this stage and ensure that what is done follows the instructions of the person, as they would have wished. And so arose, in the UK, 'Do Not Resuscitate' (DNR) orders which are now commonplace in hospitals, care homes etc. They are also referred to as 'Do Not Attempt Cardio-Pulmonary Resuscitation' or DNACPR. However it is vital that DNR orders are not used in a blanket manner for people after a certain age. Nor as has been written in the press, should anyone be coerced into signing such an order.

The obverse of properly instituted DNR orders is the gruesome attempts at resuscitation of people who have no hope of meaningful life. Some writers have referred to this as medically sanctioned 'electrocution' of dying persons, in the name of saving life.

What has all of this got to do with Covid-19? A significant proportion of people who have died from Covid-19 have been elderly and in the terminal stages of life. While every attempt should be made to make their lives comfortable and pain free, is it justifiable to attempt every possible treatment to save life? In reality it would be prolonging life until the next medical crisis. In 1901 the renowned Canadian physician Sir William Osler wrote that "pneumonia may well be called the friend of the aged. Taken off by it in an acute, short, not often painful illness, the old man escapes those 'cold gradations of decay' so distressing to himself and to his friends". Pneumonia was called the old man's friend because the person with pneumonia lapses into a state of reduced consciousness and slips away peacefully 'in their sleep, giving a dignified end to a period of often considerable suffering', according to the medical team at NetDoctor.

The same could be said of sepsis. In 2019 the Health Secretary, Matt Hancock said -"Sepsis kills over 52,000 every year— each death a preventable tragedy". But most people who die of sepsis are old, frail and at the end of life. It was reported in 2019 that 77% of sepsis related deaths in England were in people over 75 years of age. Writing in the Lancet, Dr.Mervyn Singer and his colleagues stated – 'The high incidence of frailty and severe co-morbidities makes most sepsis-related deaths neither attributable to sepsis, nor preventable through timely and effective health care.' The term 'co-morbidities' here refers to other significant illness like diabetes, coronary heart disease, heart failure, cancer etc, all of which have an adverse effect on survival.

It is therefore possible to conclude that Covid-19 was an event in the inexorable terminal journey of many people. It was the final straw, which could have been any of several other events like a stroke, heart attack, kidney failure, terminal cancer etc. It nevertheless remains important that Covid-19 be included in the death certificate. Many people for e.g. have prostate cancer but do not die of it; rather they die with it. To attribute their deaths to prostate cancer would be as erroneous as saying that all deaths in the presence of Covid-19 were due primarily to Covid-19.

Covid-19 has provided an opportunity for people and society to reflect on and talk about the care of those who are elderly, terminally ill and in the process of dying. Emma Soames, the granddaughter of Sir Winston Churchill, captured some of these concepts when she wrote 'when I depart this world I would like to have my family around me and, if I fall ill for any reason, the thought of being rushed to hospital and then dying on one's own behind a plastic curtain in an intensive care unit is not very appealing'. Peter Saul implied as much in his thought-provoking talk.

The young have been particularly badly affected by lockdown. Youthful years are the best and often the most exhilarating time of one's life, before one settles down in middle age. The young have had their education interrupted, cannot meet friends and family, and have seen their career prospects diminished. But on the whole they have accepted what had been thrown at them with a surprising graciousness - and all to protect their parents, grandparents and others of the senior generations.

The young did not suffer Covid-19 as much as their older counterparts did. Post-Covid the young generation would have difficulty with employment, and getting on the property ladder. If the latter was difficult before the pandemic it has gotten much worse after it. The young are the future of any society and the senior citizens of now owe them a debt of gratitude. If elders need to pay higher taxes to help with education, job creation and the NHS, then so be it. Children have had a particularly difficult time in lockdown being incarcerated, unable to play, to meet their friends, go to children's parties etc. Also some children and youngsters have been locked away at home with the risk of abuse. While the government was keen to protect the elderly and the NHS, it must now show that it also cares for the young and the vulnerable in society. Remember 'we are all in this together'.

While recognising the increased risks of Covid-19 and the resulting greater number of deaths from it in the BAME group of persons, governments needs to address the discrepancies. A wide ranging inquiry into the causes of the increased susceptibility and death would help focus resources where they are needed. An inquiry would include not only health and well being but also social status, education, employment, housing etc. The Marmot Review of 2010, 'Fair Society, Healthy Lives' identified several areas where improvements were needed. The report recognised that there is both a social justice case and an economic case for addressing inequalities in society. Ten years on in 2020 the Health Foundation reviewed the progress from the time of Sir Michael Marmot's report and identified widened health between wealthy and deprived areas and no improvement in life expectancy for some.

Another area of concern to the public and that needs an open honest discussion is the conflict between rights of the individual and the genuine needs of society. This conflict came into focus during the roll out of the tracing app in the UK. Concerns were raised that the app infringes human rights, especially the right to privacy. That the app is secure and was developed with privacy being paramount was ignored by some groups. There is a balance between the individual's right to privacy and the rights of the majority of people. In the case of the pandemic the right of society to be free from infection and the right of all individuals to be kept safe from the virus must be the most important principle. The app uses anonymous information to help contact others who may have the virus and so prevent spread. Lawyers who argue otherwise are putting people's lives at risk, including their own and those of their staff and families. This is the case both directly on health and indirectly from the effects on the economy of continuing infection and lockdown.

It is unfortunate that in a society like that in the UK a person may be blackballed for their views. But this is what apparently happened to two Downing Street advisers. England's Chief Nurse, Ruth May and Deputy Medical Officer, Dr Jonathan Van -Tam were both dropped from Downing Street press briefings because they public backed off from endorsing the breach of lockdown regulations by Dominic Cummings, the Prime Minister's advisor. When asked for her view on the breach at the press conference of 10th April, Ruth May responded by saying that her views were the same as those articulated by Dr.Van-Tham two days earlier when he had said ' the rules apply to all'. Although Mr. Grant Shapps MP said that Ruth May would appear at a briefing, this had not happened. While Downing Street may appear to ignore the matter, one is left with the impression that speaking truth to power is not permitted if it is against what is accepted. Everyone is the same before the law. Make exceptions and one not only generates a 'them and us' view of the matter but also the importance of the message is diluted.

The Office for National Statistics (ONS) provided the public with continuous figures of the spread of the virus in the UK, and of deaths. The daily figures also painted a picture of how effective various public health interventions were during the period of lockdown. However there was confusion in the figures provided by the ONS because initially deaths in care homes were not included in the total numbers of daily deaths. It was realised that up to a third of deaths outside of hospitals were occurring in care homes. There needs to be a clearer definition of how the prevalence of the infection is counted and also how deaths are counted. For example it would be useful to know the number of deaths directly due to Covid-19 and those deaths where the infection was an incidental or contributory factor.

A study from the Universities of Toronto and Texas casts doubt on the effectiveness of lockdown in containing Covid-19. Researchers found that richer nations were not able to reduce importation of the virus due to continuing international travel. The big advantage of lockdown was to prevent existing health services from being stretched. Earlier restriction in international travel by the UK may have reduced the numbers of cases in the country and helped improve the chances of recovery in those who got Covid-19. The biggest impact on the numbers infected was age of the population and obesity.

Researchers used the global health security (GHS) index score to assess the how countries were dealing with the epidemic and the respective outcomes in each country. GHS has six parameters to help estimate how a country is able to deal with a health threat to its population. The higher the scores for each of the parameters imply a better preparedness by the country to deal with threats to public health. Of the six parameters, that which scores the risk environment of a country and its vulnerability to biological threats was strongly associated with recovery from infections. While UK scored well against all the parameters the overall finding for all counties was that 'No country is fully prepared for epidemics or pandemics, and every country has important gaps to address'.

The pandemic has underlined, if ever it was needed, the enduring bond between the public and the NHS. The NHS is a cherished institution like no other. It is probably the greatest social experiment in the world. The pandemic has shown how much the public depend on it. Similarly, the NHS has risen to the challenge even though the lives of those who work in the NHS are at risk. The public for its part used the NHS responsibly during the crisis.

However we all know that the NHS is under-funded and yet manages to provide amazing care with the money at its disposal. The NHS has deployed new ways of working and the innovations during the epidemic are likely to last and also to change the way in which the NHS is used. Telephone and video consultations have largely met the immediate needs of patients who have bought into these new ways of communicating with doctors and other health workers. Hospital outpatient clinics have also been done remotely without, as it appears, detriment to the patient. It can be done. There is no need for large numbers of patients to attend hospital outpatient departments or GP surgeries. We have to accept the new ways of working for the benefit of all. The new normal would prevent the risk of contamination and the re-emergence of Covid-19 or any other infection.

One of the big areas of concern has been the delays to cancer care during lockdown. While it is important to maintain safety and distancing, delays in cancer care could affect health and survival. It is important, in any future pandemic or crisis of this nature that there are dedicated non – infectious hospitals. Or there has to be areas in the same hospital which are geographically separate. For e.g. patients who need chemotherapy or who have blood cancers need to have their treatments without the risk of infections. These patients should be seen in dedicated units created during planning for such eventualities. By separation of facilities, non-Covid-19 patients who need critical care like chemotherapy could have uninterrupted treatment.

A nostalgic vision of the NHS has grown in the minds and hearts of the public. This is always welcome with such a unique institution. But there are pitfalls. We should not shy away from highlighting shortfalls in the service on which all of us depend. There is the need to invest for safe and effective care. The shortage of hospital beds was been exposed by the crisis. There needs to be a minimum amount of spare capacity in every region to cope with emergencies. Also examples of less than ideal and indeed poor practice need to be highlighted. This would help the service to respond in the best way while learning lessons that can be shared by the whole organization. This should help prevent further errors and improve the quality of work.

Responsible whistle-blowing, which is still frowned upon, needs to be protected. Undue attempts to identify whistle blowers by for example taking fingerprints of staff have no place in a caring organisation. We have seen how whistle blowers provided a vital service alerting the world to the infection in China.

One area that says much about our somewhat ambivalent attitude towards the NHS is litigation. The amounts of money that the NHS is sued for are amazing. In the year 2018-2019 the amount of claims against the NHs was £9 billion. This is money that the NHS can ill afford to do without. Of course poor practices that cause people harm, interferes with gainful employment, causes death etc must in a caring society be compensated. However there are also frivolous claims where the sole purpose of the claim is to make money. Often it is easier for a hospital to settle a small claim than to go through litigation with its accompanying astronomical legal costs. The many advertisements by legal firms encouraging people to make claims do not sit well with the adulation shown to the NHS during the pandemic. There appears to be a culture of encouraging complaints for which legal firms need to take their share of responsibility. If this is curtailed, some good may result. Money saved would ultimately go towards better patient care. The public's relationship with the NHS as regards litigation needs to be reset. What better time than now.

The final words on the NHS during the pandemic must surely be about the way it coped. Compared to Italy where the health services were stretched and were often unable to cope, the NHS in the UK worked magnificently. To say otherwise is a great disservice to all those who tirelessly worked for the benefit of patients. The volunteers who helped need special mention too. There were mistakes, there are lesson to be learnt and there are policies that need to be revisited to help the UK deal with another similar crisis. The NHS may not be the best in world as some would have us believe. But in the nation's hour of need, it rose to the occasion. Even in Europe we witnessed divisions. Italy was left to its own devices, its pleas ignored while the EU allowed its member states to look after themselves. Where, one may ask, was European leadership? Was this any different with the migrant crisis or the financial crisis?

The volunteers in the NHS showed how much warmth there is for this national institution. Covid-19 also demonstrated the essential British trait of rising up to the occasion. More than 750,000 people volunteered at the country's hour of need. There is no reason to think that the same number or more would not rise up to another similar challenge if it ever came along. Covid-19 is microbiological warfare on an unprecedented level. It is rapid and it is lethal. The NHS should have its reserve 'territorial army' of volunteers to cope with any future crisis, as surely there would be.

Probably the most enduring legacies of the pandemic in the UK are likely to be the loneliness of death and the grief of absence. Loneliness in the last days of life in an intensive care unit or even in hospital or in a care home, devoid of contact with family and loved ones, must have been unbearable. The ability and freedom to say what needed to be said in the last days of a person's life and which had been left unsaid until then, must have left a painful yearning in the departed person. The same may be said of loved ones as they were separated from their nearest and dearest at the final parting. The events of Covid-19 live on in the memories of the people left behind, long after a person has departed. In this way Covid-19 is a 'watershed' in the life's journey. As the Canadian poet Anne Michelis wrote –'Grief, loss, regret are not the end of the story. They are the middle of the story.' Claire Bidwell Smith, a psychotherapist in Los Angeles, USA writes that she has seldom encountered a client who had not experienced regret after the loss of a loved one. She writes –' We cannot change our past, but we can forgive ourselves. And we can recognize that we feel this pain because we loved someone so much. And that there is endless beauty in that'.

The pandemic and lockdown has helped us to understand ourselves and our relation to each other. Each one of us has had a role in dealing with the pandemic. We needed to respect lockdown while at the same time being mindful of the needs of others. We had to look after our own health but learned the importance and effects of our acts and omissions on others. Therefore the vast majority of us acted responsibly for the greater good. We had to suspend some of the things we liked and / or wanted for e.g. going to the pub, or the theatre or the beach. Some of us may have been grudging in complying with these requests but we, nevertheless, did so because behind all of these restrictions was the safety of self and of others. Lockdown gave us a useful lesson in ethics of individual and collective responsibility and impressed upon us our interdependence on each other, nationally and internationally.

The pandemic has shown very clearly, in a way that has not been readily evident previously, how interdependent we are. Beyond the human perspective is also the realisation that we are closely linked with nature. The improvement in air quality in cities during lockdown brought home to most of us how much the planet is being polluted by human activity. We now have a chance to seize the opportunity to avoid returning to where we were in the way we lived, worked and in the balance between our needs and what we want. We can continue to look after ourselves while being mindful of the needs of others. There would be some in society who would find difficulty in accepting these simple and self-evident concepts. But as the philosopher George Wilhelm Friedrich Hegel said 'man must adhere to social needs and avoid the realities of giving in to evil.' We changed during the pandemic and lockdown; we rediscovered ourselves. We reset ourselves to what is humanity's default position As Rebecca Solnit worte in her book ' A Paradise Built in Hell: The Extraordinary Communities that Arise in Disaster', human beings are like machines that 'reset themselves to something altruistic, communitarian, resourceful and imaginative after a disaster, that we revert to something we already know how to do. The possibility of paradise is already within us as a default setting.' We have become tolerant, understanding of our neighbour and even forgiving. We have become 'each our sister's and brother's keeper.'

The cognitive revolution that allowed home sapiens to recognise and utilise intelligence has had a disastrous effect on the flora and fauna of the world. The progressive encroachment of man on the natural habitats of animals and plants has led to the gradual decimation of many species and in some instances to their eventual extinction. Covid-19 has provided a brief glimpse of what the world could be. The air in cities is cleaner, plants thrive and animals have returned to their normal habitats. Covid-19 has shown in a short period of time what Greta Thunberg, Extinction Rebellion and the like would have taken many years of protests and violence to show. We have to accept that we need to halt the decline of the planet and act responsibly to save it; we have to agree to mutually co-exist with other life forms. Could each one of us re-dedicate ourselves to becoming, even minimally, better versions of ourselves? We would then get the opportunity to preserve and enjoy the rich diversity of our planet.

We have to accept the new normal and adjust our lives to what promises to be a safer society enriched by simple values.

o0:0o

'THIS IS WAR'

The world is at war as Adayemi Mapaderun wrote in his article 'This is War' which was published in The Punch. That this is biological warfare is without doubt and we are dealing with an unseen but lethal enemy. At the time of writing there were over twenty-six million reported cases of the infection (26,622,706) world-wide. The numbers who had died the world over were more than three-quarters of a million people (874,708). In the near future it is likely that the grim milestone of one million persons dead would be passed.

In the 19th century there were over thirty wars and conflicts which caused enormous human suffering and death. This includes Word wars 1 and 2, the Vietnam War, the holocaust and the Korean War. Almost 40 million people died as a result of human conflict during these 100 years. But in that century also nearly 100 million died from the Spanish flu of 1918. Death from the flu was twice as much as from all the human conflicts of that century.

These figures give us an idea of how potent microbial warfare can be. This is in effect what the world is engaged in at present; it is likely to be a protracted microbial war. Unless the world exercises care many millions could yet die.

In any war we need to understand the enemy that we are confronted with, even though it is invisible. This would help us in our strategy for the battle ahead and with subduing and eventually overcoming our enemy- in the current context, the virus. We need to appreciate that SARS-Cov2, the virus, is an unforgiving enemy. It will exploit any and every chink in our armour to devastating effect and with fatal consequences for many. Give the virus chance and it will punish us. We only have to remember the resurgence of infections in Leicester and Greater Manchester to realize how it reared its ugly head. We need to be vigilant and this means taking all necessary precautions against the virus. We need individually and collectively to deny the virus a chance.

No one is immune from this enemy. The young may think they are immune but we need to remember what happened in the second and third waves of the Spanish flu. Large numbers of young persons died.

Unfortunately we do not have any weapons to help us prosecute this war effectively. We are passive victims of its unbridled aggression. The virus does not respect anyone. It attacks all, given a chance.

But we can limit the virus by preventing it spreading among us.

The simple steps of keeping a safe distance from others, washing our hands to prevent the virus settling on us and wearing a face covering when in a crowd are sufficient to prevent the virus infecting us.

As Mapaderun implies in his essay some or all of these actions are easier said than done. They need from all of us discipline and consistency at all times. Not doing so once may be all that the virus needs to spread.

The virus only looks for us to lower our guard. But if individually and collectively we do what is needed and deny the virus what it is seeking from us we should defeat it and return to the life of old that we yearn for.

o0:0o

ABBREVIATIONS

AGP	Aerosol Generating Procedure
BAME	Black, Asian and Minority Ethnic
C/APV	Children and Adolescent Parent Violence
CCP	Chinese Communist Party
CCS	Civil Contingencies Secretariat
CJD	Creutzfeld- Jacob disease
CMA	Competition and Markets Authority
CMO	Chief Medical Officer
CPAP	Continuous Positive Airways Pressure
CSA	Chief Scientific Advisor
CSSA	Chinese Students and Scholars Association
CTA	Common Travel Area
CQC	Care Quality Commission
ECDC	European Centre for Disease Prevention and Control
EU	European Union
FCA	Financial Conduct Authority
GDP	Gorss Domestic Product
GHS	Global Health Security index score
GP	General Practitioner (Medical)
GRG	Global Restructuring Group
HHS	US Department of Health and Human Services

HTA	Healthcare Trades Association
IMF	International Monetary Fund
LSHTM	London School of Hygiene and Tropical Medicine
MCCD	Medical Certificate of Cause of Death
MERV/ MERS	Middle Eastern Respiratory Virus / Syndrome
MP	Member of Parliament
NAO	National Audit Office
NCD	Non-communicable disease
NERVTAG	New and Emerging Respiratory Virus Threats Advisory Group
NHS	National Health Service
NICE	Nation Institute of Health and Care Excellence
NSC	National Security Council
OECD	Organisation for Economic Cooperation and Development
OfWat	Office of the Water Regulator
ONS	Office for National Statistics
PA	Professional Absenteeism
PHE	Public Health England
PHEIC	Public Health Emergency of International Concern
PM	Prime Minister
POW	Prisoner of war
PPE	Personal Protective Equipment
PPP	Pandemic Preparedness Plan
RCP	Resilience Capabilities Program
RTL	Rehabilitation Through Labour
SAGE	Scientific Advisory Group for Emergencies
SHOC	Strategic Health Operations Centre (of WHO)
SARS	Severe Acute Respiratory Syndrome
THRCC	Threats, Hazards, Resilience and Contingencies Committee
TMG	The Monitoring Group

UK	United Kingdom of Great Britain and Northern Ireland
UN	United Nations
USSR	Union of Soviet Socialist Republics
WHO	World Health Organisation
WIV	Wuhan Institute of Virology

o0:0o

www.ingramcontent.com/pod-product-compliance
Lightning Source LLC
LaVergne TN
LVHW041701060526
838201LV00043B/518